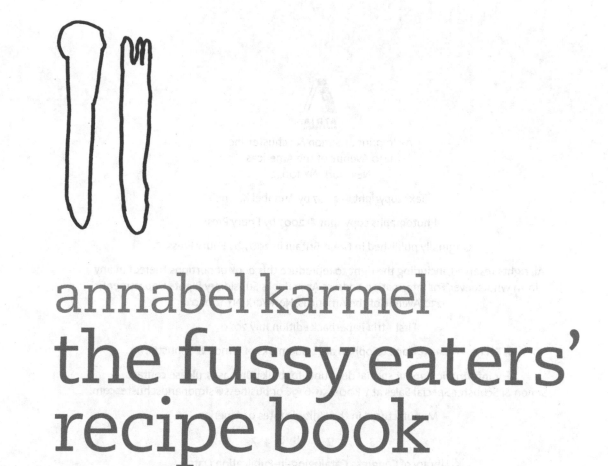

annabel karmel
the fussy eaters' recipe book

135 quick, tasty, and healthy recipes that your kids will actually eat

ATRIA PAPERBACK

New York   London   Toronto   Sydney   New Delhi

This book was inspired by fussy eaters all over the world, not least my children, Nicholas, Lara, and Scarlett.

ATRIA
PAPERBACK

An Imprint of Simon & Schuster, Inc.
1230 Avenue of the Americas
New York, NY 10020

First Atria Paperback edition July 2020

ATRIA PAPERBACK and colophon are trademarks of Simon & Schuster, Inc.

For information about special discounts for bulk purchases, please contact Simon & Schuster Special Sales at 1-800-456-6798 or business@simonandschuster.com.

Manufactured in the United States of America

1 3 5 7 9 10 8 6 4 2

Library of Congress Cataloging-in-Publication Data

Karmel, Annabel.
The fussy eaters' recipe book : 135 quick, tasty, and healthy recipes that your kids will actually eat / by Annabel Karmel.
p. cm.
Previously published: London : Ebury Press, 2007.
Includes index.
1. Quick and easy cookery.   2. Children—Nutrition.   I. Title.
TX833.5.K36   2008
641.5'55—dc22   2008021005

ISBN 978-1-4165-7876-5
ISBN 978-1-9821-5581-0 (pbk)
ISBN 978-1-4165-7881-9 (ebook)

Contents

foreword 4
top tips for fussy eaters 6
brilliant breakfasts 13
not-so-yucky vegetables 35
funky fish 65
pasta, please 89
cheeky chicken 109
mmm...eat 135
gluten-free and gorgeous 151
cookies and cakes 173
fruity finishes 199
index 218

WHAT'S THE FUSS? Anyone with children will know that when it comes to eating, fuss is often high on the menu. It's not surprising, then, that we can lose heart when our children turn their noses up at anything with green in it, or when they will allow only plain pasta with grated cheese to pass their lips! But rest assured, you're not alone. In fact, 90 percent of children go through at least one lengthy stage of being fussy. And in a 2007 survey, nearly 50 percent of parents said food was their children's worst area of fussiness, coming well ahead of clothes and even their hairstyles!

In their first year, babies grow more rapidly than at any other time in their life, so it's relatively easy to get them to eat new foods. But by the second year, your child is becoming his or her own person who'll soon figure out that refusing food is a great way of getting attention. Fortunately, nearly all children who have previously been "good eaters" do go back to eating well. The bad news, though, is that this is usually on their terms—and on their schedule.

WHY FUSS? Children's eating habits have changed dramatically in recent years. According to *The New England Journal of Medicine*, one in every three children in the United States is overweight, and one in seven is classified as obese. As a result of consuming more junk food, only two percent of children completely meet the USDA's recommendations for maintaining a healthy diet, reports a study in the journal *Pediatrics*. It doesn't have to be like this for your child.

WAVE GOOD-BYE TO FUSS! In this book, I have collected together some tasty, quick recipes to tempt the pickiest of eaters, tested by other little fusspots who've given the food the thumbs-up. For confirmed vegetable haters, you'll find cunning ways to hide the "offending items" in veggie burgers or pasta dishes. Delicious dressings will cajole your child into eating salads, and there are even great recipes for making your own healthy "junk foods" such as chicken nuggets, burgers, and pizzas.

I've also included imaginative recipes for crumbles, gelatins, and ice pops, all designed to encourage your child to eat more fruit. And there's a whole chapter on gluten-free recipes such as Polenta Mini Pizzas and Flourless Peanut Butter and Chocolate Chip Cookies so children with wheat allergies won't miss out.

By being more responsible and giving your child more home-cooked and fresh foods, you will produce meals that are healthy *and* appealing. Lifelong eating habits and tastes are formed in early childhood, and well-stocked kitchen cupboards could be your family's best form of preventive medicine.

Enjoy!

Annabel Karmel

ANNABEL KARMEL

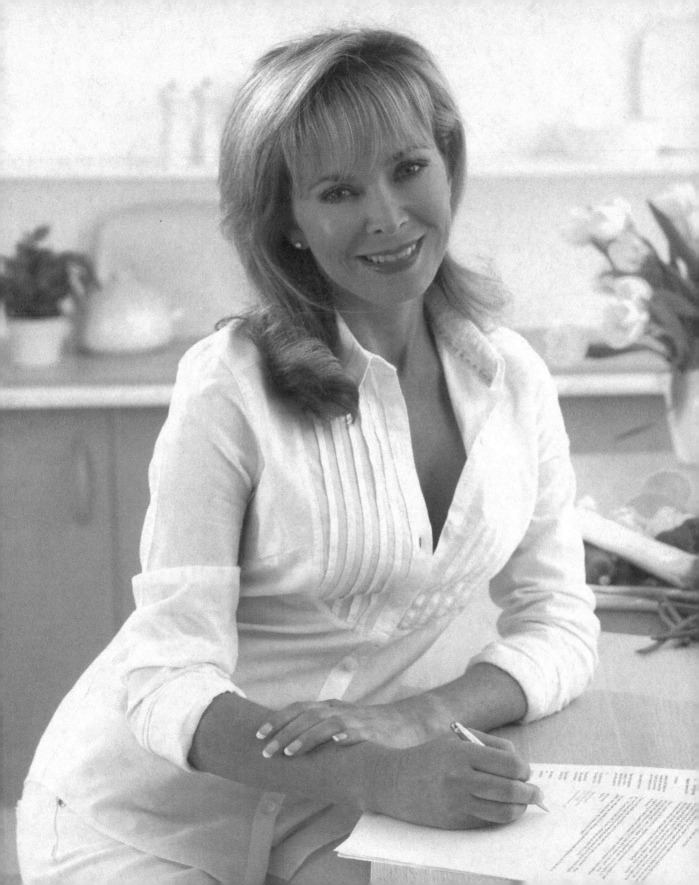

top tips
for
fussy eaters

be positive

Try to make mealtimes a really positive experience. One of the most important things is to hide your frustration. Praise your child excessively when he or she eats well or tries something new. You may need to ignore some bad eating behavior to refocus attention on good behavior. This may make mealtimes less stressful for you, too.

KIDS IN THE KITCHEN Most children adore cooking, and tasks such as squeezing fresh orange juice and cracking eggs are well within the capabilities of a young child. It's amazing how being involved in the planning and preparing of a meal can stimulate a child's appetite. Cooking is also a great way of bonding with children—spending quality time shopping for ingredients and actually making the recipes together can be a fun task for everyone involved.

It's a good idea to ask your child to invite over a group of friends, choose a menu, and get them to prepare their own lunch or supper (younger children will need a little adult supervision). Not only are they more likely to eat something they have a hand in preparing, but they are also measuring ingredients, keeping track of time, etc., all without noticing.

It's also fun to organize a cooking birthday party. Sit down with your child and choose a selection of party recipes such as Animal Cupcakes, Focaccia Pizza, My Favorite Gingersnaps, and Vegetable Kebabs. Group the children in pairs to prepare the

food. I've organized many cooking parties for my children, and they were so popular that many of their friends ended up doing the same for their birthdays.

EAT TOGETHER Eating with the whole family whenever possible can really make a difference. Personally, I think that taking the focus off your child's eating and having lots of social chat at the table is helpful. Avoid using mealtimes to assert your authority. If there is a lecture to give, choose another time.

My children are teenagers now, and on a Friday night we always try to have dinner together and take turns telling one another some of the good and bad things that happened to us during the week. Sometimes children don't realize that bad things happen to adults, too, so it doesn't matter whether it's trivial or important— dinnertime is a time for communicating and getting to know one another. It can soon become a regular family ritual. Children are more likely to open up to you if you are open with them, and it's good bonding time.

REWARD SCHEMES In a recent survey, 25 percent of mothers said that they dread mealtimes, and nearly 50 percent admitted they resort to bribery to get their children to eat up. Sticker charts usually work best once your child reaches two and a half. Keep portions absolutely minuscule (your child can always ask for more and will get a sense of achievement for finishing his or her meal), and at first give a sticker for just trying the food. Your child could have a yogurt as a reward for trying his or her main course. The treats for completing a sticker chart should not be unhealthy foods (e.g., sweets), as this gives the wrong message. Ideally, they should be small and affordable (you may be doing sticker charts for quite a long time!). Make the charts yourself, perhaps using pictures of your child's favorite things (tractors, fairies, etc.) to decorate it. You could even download pictures from the Internet for your child to color in to make the sticker chart with you. Try to keep them short for this age group so that the first one is relatively easily attainable and teaches your child the purpose of these charts.

Another useful reward scheme, for slightly older children, is to fill an empty jar with small objects such as dried pasta shapes. One pasta shape is awarded for eating a meal or trying something new (or any other good behavior). Start with a small jar and let your child put the pasta in him- or herself. A small present or treat (e.g., family trip to beach/football game/ Rollerblading in the park) is the prize for filling the jar so that the lid does not fit on.

Encourage your child to make an "Eat Up" book. Buy a scrapbook and get your child to stick in the packaging or a photo of the new food that he or she eats. You could find some old food magazines and cut out photos of foods that you would like to get your child to eat and keep them in a shoe box. You could also get your child to draw pictures of the new food. Each time your child has tried or eaten six new foods and stuck them in the book, he or she gets a reward. It might be stickers, jewelry, sports equipment, or a trip to the movies—choose something that would appeal to your child and isn't too expensive.

tea Parties

Invite your child's friends to tea—especially if they are good eaters—so that your child can see his or her friends eating happily. This also helps to keep meals fun and sociable.

don't make a fuss

If your child refuses to eat anything other than junk food, chill out. He or she will soon find there's not much point making a fuss if you don't react.

MAKE FOOD ATTRACTIVE AND FUN

Give small portions—it's not good to overload your child's plate. Also, children generally prefer smaller pieces of food, so it's a good idea to make foods such as mini burgers with baby potatoes, small broccoli florets, and mini carrots. They also like eating from small containers, so use ramekins to prepare individual portions of foods. You can also make a batch and freeze them.

Attractive presentation can make the difference between your child's accepting and refusing food. Whole fruit may not get eaten, but thread bite-size fresh fruit onto skewers or straws and it immediately becomes more appealing.

Children also like to assemble their own food, so you could lay ingredients out in bowls and let your children fill and fold their own wraps or choose their favorite toppings for their homemade pizzas.

BLIND MAN'S GRUB

If you have a little "junk food junkie" who refuses to try anything new, play a game in which you blindfold your child and give her several foods to taste, some old favorites and some new, and see if she can identify what they are.

HEALTHY JUNK FOOD

Create your own "healthy junk food." Make pizza bases using mini bagels, English muffins, focaccia bread, or pita bread and let your child choose his or her favorite toppings. Make burgers using good-quality lean beef—and I have my own delicious version of chicken nuggets, for which you marinate the chicken in buttermilk, soy sauce, Worcestershire sauce, paprika, and lemon and then coat in bread crumbs and Parmesan.

START AS YOU MEAN TO CONTINUE

Start your baby off on fresh baby food rather than jars of processed food with a shelf life of two years. If they are used to a variety of fresh flavors early on, children are much less likely to become fussy eaters when you try to integrate fresh foods into family meals.

Once a child's palate has become accustomed to the intense sweetness of refined sugary foods, it is harder for him or her to appreciate the more gentle natural sweetness of fruit. If you want your child to enjoy fresh fruit, restrict sugary foods.

HEALTHY SNACKS After school is a great time to get your child to eat something healthy, as they generally come home starving. The trouble is that most children dive into the cookie jar or grab a chocolate bar after school. Have something ready prepared on the table. Cut-up fruit on a plate is much more tempting than fruit in a fruit bowl, and children like raw veggies with a tasty dip. It's quick and easy to make delicious wraps, pita pockets, or pasta salads, and it's a good idea to have a low shelf in the fridge from which children can help themselves to tasty healthy snacks.

Reduce snacks between meals to one in the morning and one in the afternoon and make sure they are healthy.

Try to control how much—and what—your child drinks between meals and at mealtimes. Try to encourage him or her to drink more water.

YOUR DENTIST IS YOUR ALLY Next time you go, ask the dentist to explain to your child what will happen to his teeth if he eats too many sweets and drinks too many sugary drinks. You can remind him of this the next time he demands the latest sweets he has seen on TV. Limit sweets to once or twice a week.

LET THEM PACK THEIR OWN LUNCH Get your child involved in packing his own lunch box—that way you will know what foods he finds acceptable. There are some foods children may eat at home but won't eat in front of friends. Also make sure food is easy and quick to eat. Children won't bother with anything complicated because they are usually in a rush to get to the playground. If you give fruit, it's usually best to cut it up or peel fruits such as clementines and wrap them in plastic wrap.

CHANGE OF SCENERY Take food outdoors in the summer and have a picnic. This could just be in the backyard. For some children, a change of scenery works wonders. You could even take teddy bears and spare plates and cups so that the bears can "eat" with you.

In the summer, barbecues tend to be popular with children—they like hamburgers, drumsticks, or corn on the cob cooked on the barbecue.

It's also fun to play make-believe if children are preparing a meal themselves. Let them create a restaurant in one of the rooms in your house. My children used to love doing this: one would be the waiter, the other the chef.

eating out

Watch out for kids' menus in restaurants—they often read like a fast-food menu. Ask for a half portion from the adult menu instead. Compliment your child on behaving like a grown-up—children's taste in food is more sophisticated than you might imagine.

variety is the spice of life

Do not just stick to favorite meals. Offer a variety of healthy dishes and keep trying new recipes. Offering only the foods that you are sure your child will eat can encourage extreme fussiness and may lead to a restricted and unbalanced diet.

TRY SOMETHING NEW You are probably frustrated when children refuse to eat something that they have never even tasted. A fear of new foods is known as neophobia. It generally develops at around eighteen months, and babies who would happily accept many foods suddenly become suspicious and reject anything unfamiliar. If your child has a very restricted diet, it is best to give new foods when she is really hungry, let her see other people eating the same food, try to encourage her to eat just a small amount, and give lots of attention and praise if she is willing to try it. If she still refuses to eat it, maybe mix it together with something she likes. For example, if your child likes pasta but won't eat vegetables, try making a lasagne with spinach.

DON'T BE SCARED OF SAYING NO Children are good at inducing parental guilt, but you will make your life difficult if they know that they can twist you around their little fingers. Instead of rewarding good behavior with sweets, encourage children to choose treats such as stickers or comics.

PLAY THE FOOD DETECTIVE GAME Make rejecting unhealthy food into a game—ask your child to find a drink that contains less than 10 percent juice, and then get him to look for one with the words "pure fruit juice" or "100 percent juice." Ask your child to find you a breakfast cereal that isn't high in salt or sugar by picking a cereal with less than 300mg sodium per serving and no added sugar.

If your child pesters you to buy something, ask him to read the ingredients list, and if there is a long list of additives that he can't pronounce because he doesn't know what they are, don't buy it.

GIVE YOUR CHILD A CHOICE Talk to your child about what he or she likes and dislikes and what he or she might want for supper in the coming week. Involving your child will lead to less conflict over food.

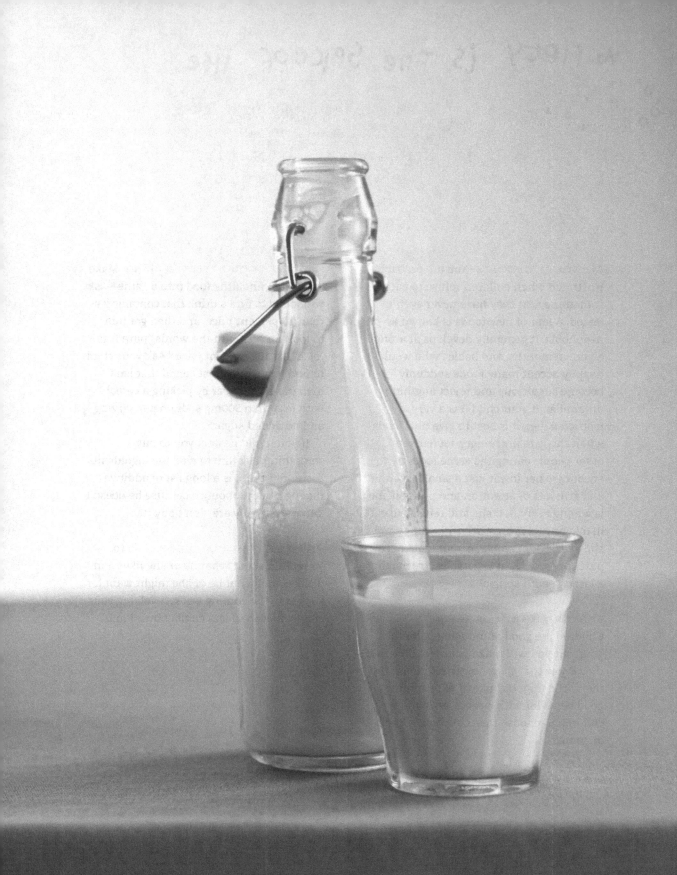

brilliant
breakfasts

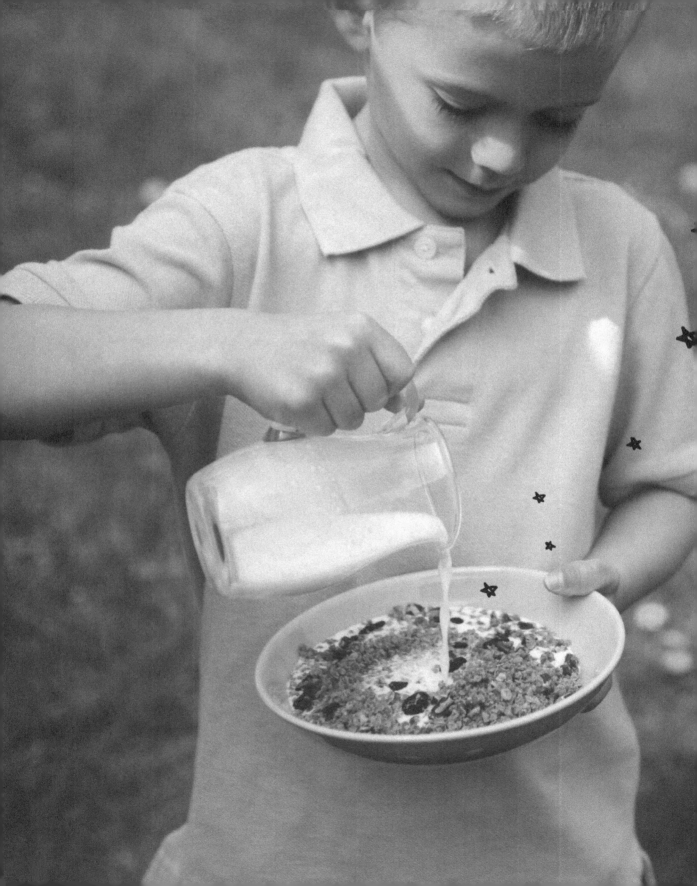

how to get your child to eat a good breakfast

* Try not to buy sugary refined cereals—it's much more difficult to get your child to enjoy healthy cereals once he is used to a sweet taste. Choose instead slow-burning carbohydrates for long-lasting energy, such as shredded wheat, muesli, oatmeal, or whole wheat toast.

* A bowl of cereal is a healthy start to the day, but you will need to choose carefully. Many cereals aimed at children contain more than 40 percent sugar. It's easy to make your own Fruity Muesli or delicious granola (see pages 17 and 19).

* When your child's iron stores are low, less oxygen gets to the brain, resulting in difficulty in concentrating and a shortened attention span. Breakfast cereals are a good source of iron, but you need to give your child vitamin C with his cereal—for example, a glass of orange juice or some strawberries or kiwifruit. He needs vitamin C to be able to absorb the iron in the cereal.

* Smoothies are good for breakfast, and your child will enjoy making these himself.

* Eggs are good for breakfast—whether it's a scrambled egg, French toast, or a soft-boiled egg with toast.

* Get most of it ready the night before so that you are not stressed in the morning.

* Don't let your child skip breakfast. If your child claims not to be hungry first thing or there is no time to fit in breakfast, think back to the previous evening. When did he last eat and what time did he go to bed? The earlier your child eats and the earlier he goes to bed, the more likely it is that he will want food first thing and the easier it will be to get him up fifteen minutes earlier.

* Try to eat breakfast with your child if you can.

* A good breakfast should contain some protein (e.g., eggs, cheese, or yogurt), whole-grain cereal or bread, and some fresh fruit.

* Be flexible—my children have been known to eat odd things for breakfast, such as mini muffin pizzas or tomato soup. Something from last night's dinner might tempt them more than a bowl of cereal. As long as it's nutritious, it doesn't really matter what it is.

* If your child has to get to school early and just doesn't have time for breakfast, you can make delicious fruit muffins that he could eat on his way to school with a fruit smoothie.

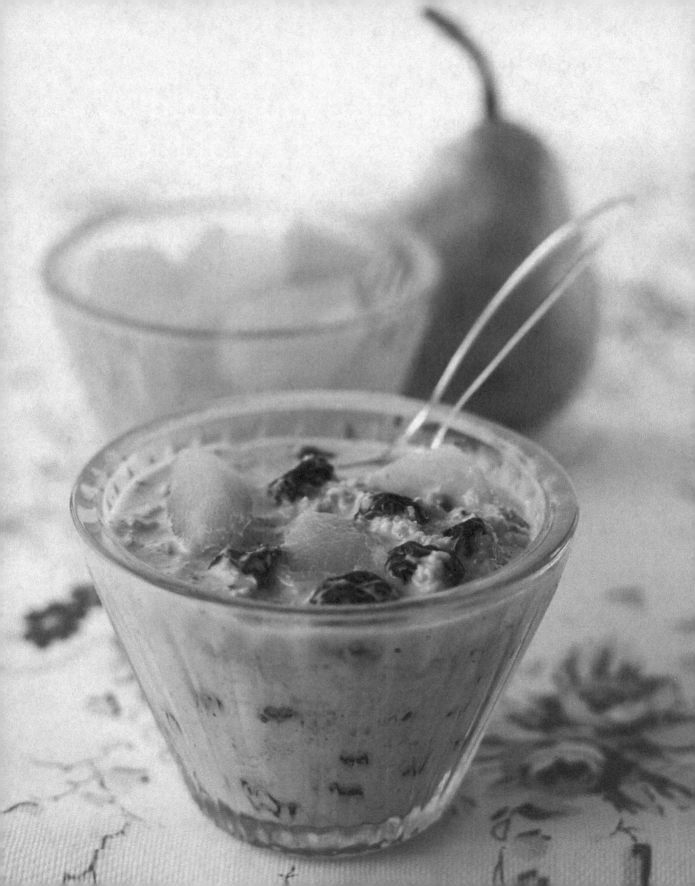

fruity muesli

A Swiss-style muesli is a good way to encourage children to eat oats, especially if they are not keen on "gloppy" oatmeal. If your child is particularly fussy, then try substituting her favorite fruit yogurt for the plain yogurt.

3 tablespoons quick-cooking oats
2 tablespoons orange juice or apple juice
2 tablespoons plain yogurt
½ small apple, peeled, cored, and grated
1 tablespoon milk
1 teaspoon honey

SUGGESTED TOPPINGS
APRICOT AND STRAWBERRY
2 dried apricots, chopped
2 strawberries, quartered
GRAPE AND BLUEBERRY
3 seedless grapes, halved
1 tablespoon blueberries
PEACH
1 juicy ripe peach, peeled and chopped

* Soak the oats overnight in the fridge in a mixture of the orange juice or apple juice and yogurt.
* In the morning, stir in the grated apple, milk, and honey. Then add fruits of your choice.

☆ The best way to deliver long-lasting energy in the morning is to give your child complex carbohydrates such as whole wheat bread, or whole-grain cereals such as oats, and fruit. The fiber contained in these foods helps slow down the rate at which sugar is released, giving increased concentration and sustained energy. It's easy to make your own delicious mueslis by soaking oats overnight and then mixing in fruits of your choice in the morning.

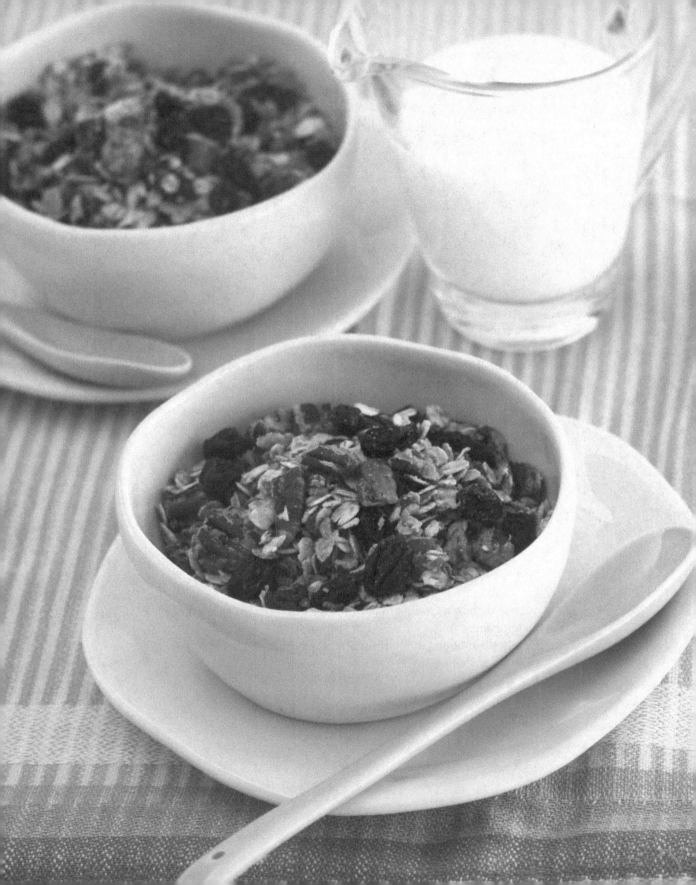

annabel's granola

This delicious granola is very versatile. You can have it for breakfast with milk. It's also very good on its own as a snack or layered with yogurt, honey, and fruit. If your child is anti-nuts or allergic, then you could substitute pumpkin seeds instead, or double the quantity of raisins.

2 cups quick-cooking oats
½ cup coarsely chopped pecans
¼ cup unsweetened flaked coconut
¼ teaspoon salt
¼ cup packed light brown sugar
2 tablespoons canola oil
¼ cup maple syrup
½ cup raisins

* Preheat the oven to 300°F. Put the oats, pecans, coconut, salt, and sugar in a large bowl and mix with a wooden spoon.
* Whisk the oil and maple syrup together in a small bowl. Pour over the oats and mix well.
* Spread out on a lightly oiled baking sheet and bake in the center of the oven for 40 to 45 minutes, stirring every 10 minutes.
* Transfer to a bowl, stir in the raisins, and leave to cool.

☆ Whole-grain cereals are a good source of iron. However, it is difficult for our bodies to absorb iron from a nonmeat source (red meat provides the most easily absorbed form of iron). To improve the absorption of iron from breakfast cereal, you need to give your child vitamin C–rich fruit, such as kiwifruit or berries, or vitamin C–rich juice, such as orange or cranberry juice.

almost instant oatmeal

Soaking the oats overnight speeds up the cooking time and makes this a fast but very nutritious breakfast. Fussy eaters should be tempted by one of the delicious toppings.

3 tablespoons quick-cooking oats
⅔ cup milk

* Soak the oats overnight in the milk in the fridge.
* In the morning, put in a microwavable bowl and cook for 1 minute on high. Stir, then cook for 30 seconds or until just boiling (lower-wattage microwaves may need 30 seconds more). Stir again, thoroughly, and allow to cool slightly before serving. (Remember that more than one portion will take longer to cook.)
* Alternatively, transfer the oats to a pan and bring to a boil, stirring. Allow to cool slightly before serving.

SUGGESTED TOPPINGS

BANANA AND MAPLE SYRUP
½ small banana, sliced
2 teaspoons maple syrup

APPLE, CINNAMON, AND RAISIN
a generous knob of butter
1 small apple, peeled and chopped
1 tablespoon raisins
2 teaspoons light brown sugar
a pinch of ground cinnamon
* Melt the butter in a pan and sauté the chopped apple with the raisins, brown sugar, and cinnamon for 2 to 3 minutes.

APRICOT AND HONEY
3 dried apricots, diced
1 to 2 teaspoons honey

CRUNCHY STRAWBERRY
2 or 3 strawberries, diced
1 to 2 teaspoons turbinado sugar or granulated sugar

omelet crepe

A thin omelet can be a less challenging way for children to eat eggs in the morning, particularly if you add some of their favorite fillings.

1 large egg
2 tablespoons milk
salt and freshly ground black pepper, to season
1 teaspoon butter
a small handful of grated Cheddar

* Beat the egg and milk together thoroughly with a little salt and pepper.
* Warm an 8-inch nonstick frying pan over medium heat, add the butter, and, once melted, pour in the egg mixture and swirl to cover the base. Cook for about 1 minute until starting to set. Sprinkle the cheese and filling of your choice on top (see below). Cook for another 2 minutes, then slip onto a plate and carefully roll up.

SUGGESTED FILLINGS
½ large tomato, seeded and diced
1 small scallion, sliced
3 mushrooms, sliced and sautéed in 1 teaspoon butter or oil
crumbled slice of cooked bacon
1 slice ham, diced (and optional ½ diced tomato)
2 tablespoons cooked chicken, chopped, and ½ diced tomato
2 tablespoons drained canned corn, ½ diced tomato, and a small scallion, sliced
1 tablespoon finely diced red bell pepper
1 slice smoked salmon, cut into thin strips

☆ A list of the nutritional content of eggs reads like a who's who of healthy nutrients. They are rich in protein and zinc and vitamins A, D, E, and B_{12} (the latter is essential for vegetarians, as eggs are one of the few nonmeat sources of this vitamin). Egg yolks contain lecithin, thought to be an important "brain food" that contributes to memory and concentration. The yolks also contain iron, which is vital for good brain function.

i don't like...

milk unless it's a chocolate milkShake

berry burst

Most children love summer fruits, but if they find the seeds off-putting, then pass the blended smoothie through a strainer before serving.

½ cup fresh or frozen summer berries
1 small banana, cut into chunks
3 tablespoons strawberry yogurt
2 teaspoons honey
¼ cup cold milk

* If using frozen fruits, leave them to thaw for about 20 minutes. Put the berries, banana, yogurt, and honey into a blender and whiz for 1 to 2 minutes, until smooth. Add the milk and whiz again until frothy.
* Pour into a glass to serve.

sunshine smoothie

This smoothie is a great way to use up slightly overripe bananas—the ones with brown spots that children hate to eat.

1 medium banana, cut into chunks
½ large mango, peeled and cut into chunks
1 teaspoon honey
½ cup pineapple juice
¼ cup orange juice

* Put the banana, mango, and honey into a blender and whiz for 1 to 2 minutes, until smooth. Add the pineapple juice and orange juice and whiz again until frothy.
* Pour into a glass to serve.

Strawberries ☺ and cream

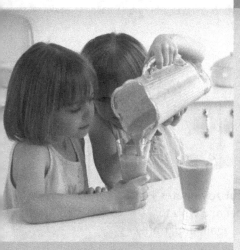

TIP
Smoothies are a great way not only to tempt fussy eaters to have a nutritious breakfast but also to hide the fact that you are giving them a couple of portions of fruit!

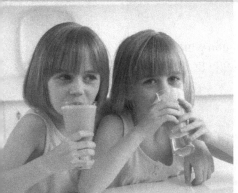

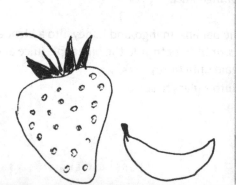

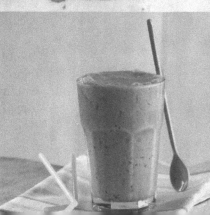

strawberries and cream

The cream soda adds a delicious flavor
to this smoothie. It's one of my favorites.

1 medium banana, cut into chunks
5 to 8 medium strawberries, halved
3 tablespoons strawberry yogurt
¼ cup cream soda

* Put the banana, strawberries, and yogurt
into a blender and whiz for 1 to 2 minutes,
until smooth. Add the cream soda
and whiz again until frothy.
* Pour into a glass to serve.

bananarama

For a banana-split smoothie, use chocolate
syrup instead of maple syrup. You could use
all milk if you prefer.

1 medium banana, cut into chunks
3 tablespoons vanilla yogurt
1 tablespoon maple syrup
¼ cup apple juice
2 tablespoons cold milk

* Put the banana, yogurt, and maple syrup
into a blender and whiz for 1 to 2 minutes,
until smooth. Add the apple juice and milk
and whiz again until frothy.
* Pour into a glass to serve.

grace's dairy-free summer berry smoothie

Tofu is soybean curd made from soy
milk. It provides a good source of calcium,
so adding it to smoothies if your child has
a cow's milk allergy is a good idea. There are
two types of tofu—firm tofu and the silken
tofu that I have used in this recipe.

1 pound fresh or frozen summer berries
½ cup small chunks silken tofu
2 cups cold soy milk
1 to 2 tablespoons honey

* If using frozen berries, leave them
to thaw for about 20 minutes. Put the
berries into a blender. Add the tofu, soy
milk, and honey to taste and blend until
smooth and creamy.
* Pour into 4 glasses and serve
immediately.

french toast with caramelized apples

Challah, a braided yeast bread made with eggs, is traditionally served on Friday night in Jewish households, and is good for making French toast. Use slightly stale challah, or brioche, a good alternative. Instead of caramelized apples, try blueberry compote: put ⅔ cup blueberries in a pan; add 1 tablespoon superfine sugar and a squeeze of lemon juice. Heat gently until the blueberries pop open and release their juices, and then simmer for 2 to 3 minutes.

CARAMELIZED APPLES
1 tablespoon unsalted butter
2 tablespoons superfine sugar
2 medium apples, peeled, cored, and cut into 12 wedges

FRENCH TOAST
2 thick slices slightly stale challah or white bread, crusts removed
2 eggs
2 tablespoons milk
1½ teaspoons superfine sugar
3 or 4 drops vanilla extract
a knob of butter, for frying
a pinch of ground cinnamon, for sprinkling

* For the apples, melt the butter in a frying pan over medium heat. Stir in the sugar until dissolved. Add the apple slices and, turning them occasionally, cook for 5 to 10 minutes until soft and just turning golden.
* Cut the bread into novelty shapes like animals or hearts, using cookie cutters, or simply cut into sticks or triangles. Beat the eggs with the milk, ¾ teaspoon of the sugar, and the vanilla and pour into a shallow dish. Heat a frying pan over medium heat and add the butter. Soak the bread in the beaten egg, then fry each piece for 2 to 3 minutes on each side, until golden.
* Mix the remaining ¾ teaspoon sugar and the cinnamon together and sprinkle over the hot French toast. Serve the caramelized apples on the side.

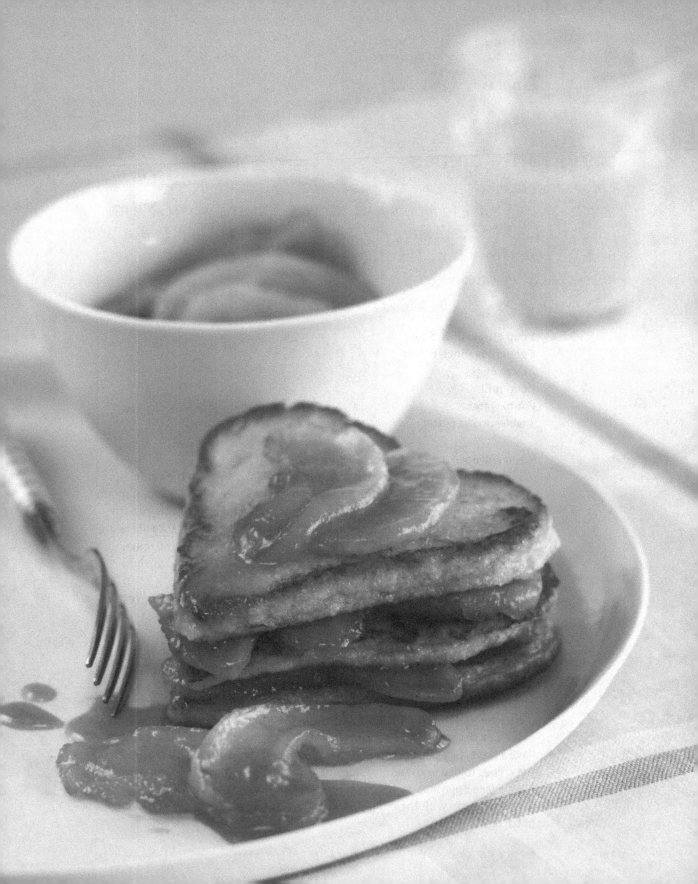

my favorite crepes

Crepes for breakfast are a real treat and you can make delicious, really thin crepes with this foolproof batter. Sprinkle them with fresh lemon juice and dust with confectioners' sugar or serve with maple syrup and perhaps some fresh fruit. These crepes would also make a wonderful dessert or after-school treat.

1 cup all-purpose flour
a generous pinch of salt
2 large eggs
1 cup milk
½ cup water
3 tablespoons butter

* You will need a heavy-bottomed 8-inch skillet or crepe pan.
* Sift the flour and salt into a large mixing bowl. Make a well in the center and crack in the eggs. Beat them into the flour using a whisk or a wooden spoon.
* In a separate bowl, mix the milk and water, then gradually beat this into the egg-and-flour mixture until the batter is smooth with the consistency of cream.
* Melt the butter and stir 2 tablespoons of it into the batter. Pour the remaining 1 tablespoon butter into a bowl. Scrunch up some paper towels and dip into the butter.
* Use the buttery paper to smear the bottom of the crepe pan. Always get the pan really hot before pouring in the batter and then turn down the heat to medium. If the first crepe sticks, it's because the pan isn't hot enough. You will need about 2 tablespoons of batter for each crepe, and it is a good idea to pour this into a ladle so that it goes into the pan in one go. Tilt the pan quickly until the bottom is covered with a thin layer of batter.
* Cook over medium heat for about 1 minute until you can see the pan through the batter and the edges begin to lift. Slide a spatula under the crepe and flip it over. Cook the second side for about 30 seconds. The first side of the crepe should have a pretty lacy pattern, while the second side will be spotted with brown. Serve the crepes folded with the lacy side out and one of your favorite toppings and fillings (see opposite).
* Wipe the pan with the re-dipped buttery paper before adding the next ladleful of batter.

FAVORITE CREPE TOPPINGS AND FILLINGS

LEMON AND SUGAR The classic fresh-lemon-juice-and-sugar combination is hard to beat. Squeeze some fresh lemon juice on top and a sprinkling of superfine sugar and then fold in half.

CHOCOLATE For chocolate lovers, smooth melted chocolate, or chocolate spread, over the crepes. It's also good to add peeled chopped pears. Fold the crepes over and then drizzle with some ready-made chocolate sauce.

PEACH MELBA Spread each crepe with a little strawberry or raspberry jam, add a few chopped well-drained canned or fresh peach slices, and fold the crepes in half. Top each with a scoop of vanilla ice cream.

MAPLE SYRUP Crepes topped with a scoop of vanilla ice cream and then drizzled with warm maple syrup are delicious.

CARAMELIZED APPLE Use the recipe for French Toast with Caramelized Apples (page 26).

TOFFEE BANANA

4 tablespoons (½ stick) butter
¼ cup packed light brown sugar
3 tablespoons heavy cream
2 tablespoons golden syrup, such as Lyle's, or light corn syrup
4 small bananas, sliced
vanilla ice cream, to serve

* To make the toffee sauce, place the butter, sugar, cream, and golden syrup in a pan. Heat gently until melted, then bring to a boil and let bubble for 1 minute. Spoon some sliced banana onto one side of each crepe, drizzle some of the sauce on top, fold in half, and then spoon some more of the toffee sauce on top and serve with a scoop of vanilla ice cream.

☆ You can make the crepes in advance and freeze them or store them in the fridge for a couple of days, interleaved with baking parchment and covered with plastic wrap. To reheat, preheat the oven to 350°F. Stack the crepes on a heatproof plate and cover with foil. Warm in the oven for 10 to 15 minutes. To microwave, stack, cover with plastic wrap, pierce the wrap, and reheat on high for 1 minute. You will need to increase these times if reheating from frozen.

raisin bran breakfast muffins

Muffins are good, as your child can take them with him if he got up late and didn't have time for breakfast. I have used whole wheat flour to maximize the fiber content in these muffins, but feel free to use half whole wheat and half all-purpose if you prefer (reduce the milk by a couple of tablespoons).

1½ cups raisin bran cereal, plus extra for topping
1 cup milk, warmed
1 heaping cup whole wheat flour
2 teaspoons baking powder
¼ teaspoon salt
1 teaspoon ground cinnamon
½ teaspoon ground ginger
½ cup raisins
1 large egg
½ cup packed dark brown sugar
½ cup canola oil
2 tablespoons turbinado or raw sugar, for topping

* Preheat the oven to 400°F. Line a muffin pan with 8 paper cases.
* Put the cereal in a bowl with the milk and leave to stand for 5 minutes or until the cereal is soft (this can sit while you measure out the other ingredients).
* Combine the flour, baking powder, salt, and spices in a large bowl. Stir in the raisins. Beat together the egg, brown sugar, and oil and add to the flour mixture, along with the soaked cereal and any milk left in the bowl. Mix.
* Spoon the batter into the muffin cases (fill to the top). Crush a small handful of flakes from the extra raisin bran, combine with the turbinado sugar, and sprinkle over the muffins. Bake for 20 to 25 minutes until risen and firm to the touch. Allow to cool for 5 minutes in the pan, then transfer to a wire rack to cool completely.
* Store in an airtight container for up to 5 days.

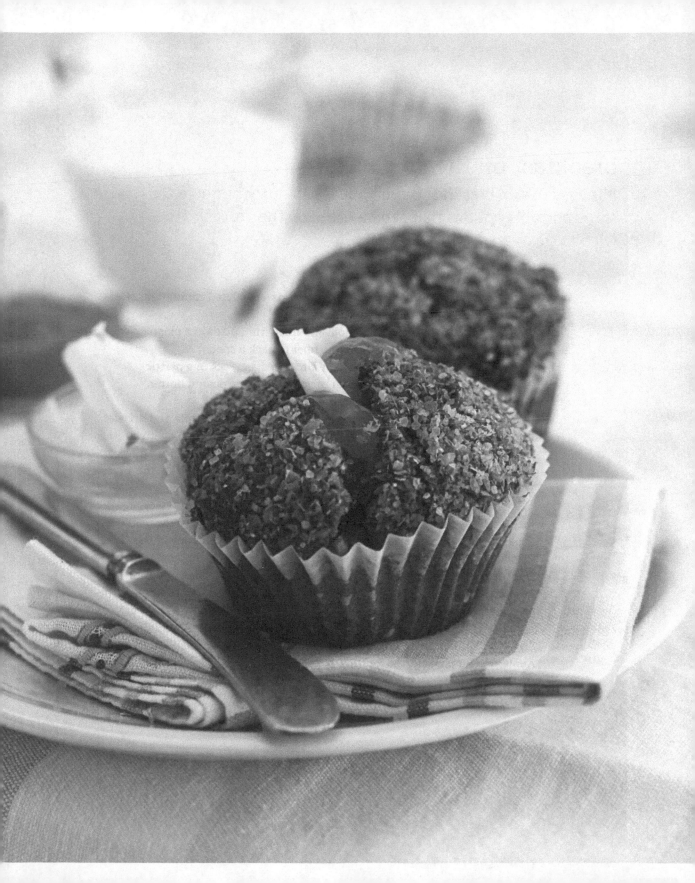

breakfast on the go

It is easy to skip breakfast if everyone is in a hurry, but here are some portable options that can be eaten on the go. Pack a wet wipe to clean up sticky fingers!

SMOOTHIES in plastic cups with screw-top lids—insulated commuter coffee mugs are ideal. Shake well before drinking.

GRANOLA Alternate layers of granola and fresh fruit; place in a plastic container with a tight-fitting lid. Remember to pack a spoon.

FRUIT DIPPERS Core an apple and cut into 8 wedges. Pack in a plastic sandwich bag with a small container of yogurt or some peanut butter. Dip the apple in the yogurt or peanut butter.

FRUIT WRAP Spread 1½ tablespoons cream cheese over a tortilla and drizzle 1 teaspoon of honey on top. Put ½ sliced banana at one end along with a few blueberries or a couple of sliced strawberries or 1 tablespoon of diced mango. Roll up and wrap in foil. The foil can be peeled off as your child eats the wrap. This filling is also good in a sandwich made with whole-grain bread.

BREAKFAST WRAP Melt 2 teaspoons of butter in a small pan. Beat 2 eggs with 1 tablespoon of milk and a little salt and pepper and add to the pan. Cook, stirring over low heat, until the egg has scrambled. Add any of the following to the scrambled egg: ham, bacon, grated cheese, chopped tomato, smoked salmon, sautéed diced bell pepper and onion plus a few drops of Tabasco. Pile onto one side of a tortilla and roll up. Wrap in foil. The foil can be peeled off as your child eats the wrap.

FRUIT MUFFINS are perfect for eating on the way to school, as are Raisin Bran Breakfast Muffins (page 30), Jamaican Banana Muffins (page 181), and Oat, Apple, and Sunflower Seed Muffins (page 183).

i don't like . . .

egg

a ny way at all

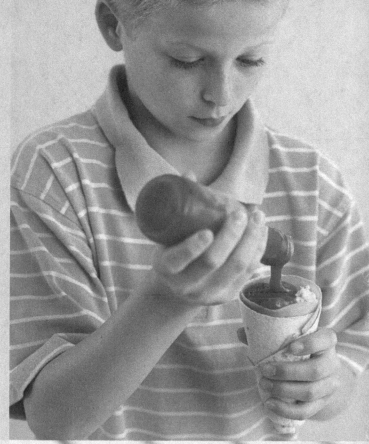

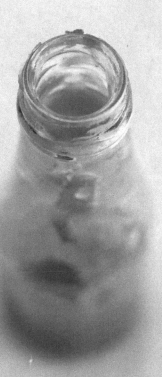

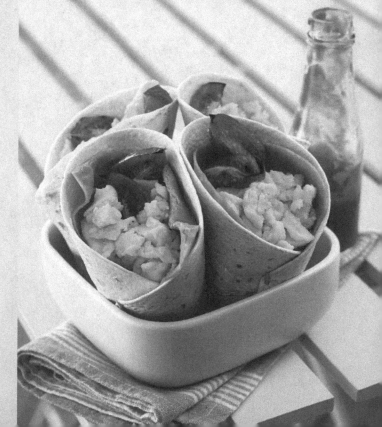

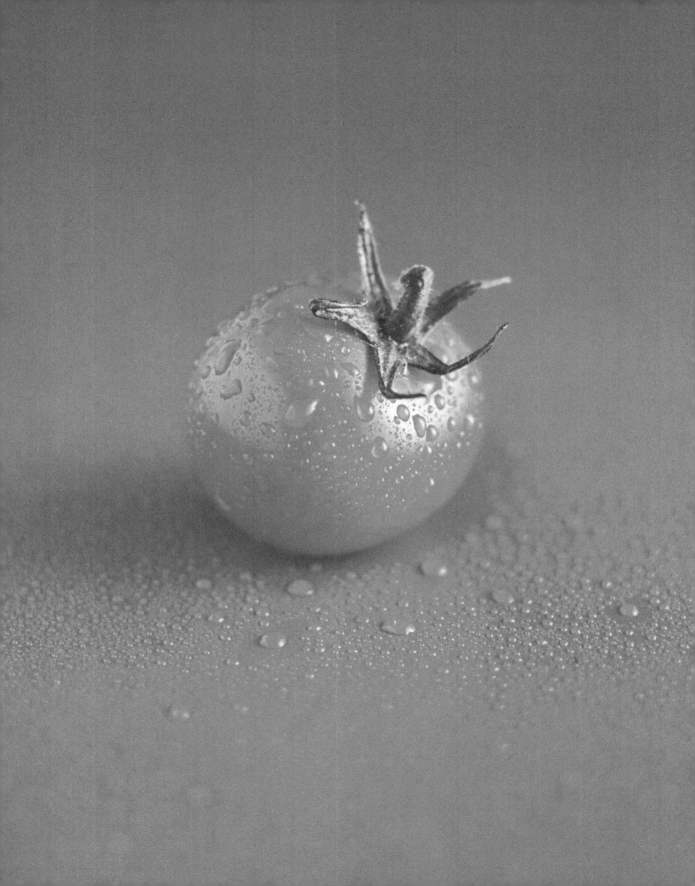

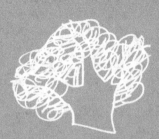

Not-so-yucky vegetables

top tips

how to get your child to eat vegetables

* Offer veggie sticks. Many children who don't like cooked vegetables will eat them raw. Vegetables such as carrot, cucumber, and bell pepper sticks make great snacks any time of the day and you can serve them with a tasty dip like hummus.

* Disguise vegetables by blending them into a tomato sauce and serve with pasta. You can double-bluff by leaving a few chunky vegetables in the sauce for your child to pick out, then he'll never suspect that there are still some in there.

* Overcooked soggy vegetables are a turn-off. Steam rather than boil vegetables: they taste and look better. Alternatively, stir-fry vegetables. It's worth buying a wok—stir-frying snow peas in a little butter is much nicer than boiling them.

* You can sneak vegetables into other popular dishes such as wraps, cannelloni, lasagne, or quesadillas, or hide vegetables under grated cheese in pizzas.

* A simple batter can transform vegetables into an exciting snack. If you can't get your child to eat any green vegetables, try making zucchini sticks with a crispy coating flavored with Parmesan. How about growing your own vegetables and getting your child involved? It's surprisingly easy to grow vegetables such as potatoes, broccoli, zucchini, and green beans. Children will be intrigued to eat something they have grown themselves.

* Instead of boring mashed potatoes, why not combine mashed potatoes with carrot or sweet potato—it's a good source of beta-carotene. Sweet potato is also delicious on its own and contains more vitamins and fiber than ordinary potato. You can use it as a substitute for potato to make oven-baked potato wedges or you can mash them. Interestingly, the more colorful the vegetable, the better it is for you, as the pigment contains valuable antioxidants.

* The secret to getting your child to enjoy eating salad is to come up with a delicious dressing. There are some yummy dressings in this book and clever ways with salads, like adding crispy noodles or giving the salad a Japanese flavor by adding mirin, soy sauce, rice wine vinegar, and honey.

* Try adding some more unusual vegetables like napa cabbage, snow peas, and bean sprouts to stir-fries. Add a splash of teriyaki sauce and some noodles for added child appeal. And how about some child-friendly chopsticks that are joined at the top—your child will have so much fun picking up the food, he will forget to make a fuss.

* Children like eating with their fingers, so serve vegetables such as corn on the cob with melted butter, or baked potato wedges.

butternut squash risotto

Rice and pasta dishes tend to be popular with fussy children, so it's a good idea to combine these with nutritious ingredients. Butternut squash is very rich in vitamin A, which is important for healthy skin, eyesight, and fighting infection.

1 medium butternut squash, peeled, seeded, and cut into ½-inch cubes
2 tablespoons olive oil
salt and freshly ground black pepper, to season
2 tablespoons butter
1 large shallot or small onion, diced
1 garlic clove, crushed
1 cup risotto rice (such as arborio)
about 5¼ cups hot vegetable or chicken broth
¼ cup freshly grated Parmesan, plus extra to serve
1 tablespoon heavy cream
1½ teaspoons chopped fresh parsley or a little chopped fresh sage, to serve
(optional)

* Preheat the oven to 400°F.
* Toss the squash in the oil and a little salt and pepper, then spread out
on a nonstick baking sheet. Roast for 20 minutes, turning halfway through.
* Melt the butter in a 3-quart saucepan and gently cook the shallot or onion for
5 minutes, or until soft but not colored. Add the garlic and rice and cook for
2 minutes, or until the rice starts to turn translucent. Add 1½ cups of the hot
broth (keeping the broth hot throughout) and bring to a simmer, stirring. Leave
to cook for 5 minutes, then add another 1½ cups broth and stir well. Simmer for
another 5 minutes, then add 1 cup broth and stir well again. Simmer for another
8 to 10 minutes, until the rice is tender.
* Add the roasted squash and the Parmesan with another 1 cup broth and cook,
stirring, for another 2 minutes. Stir in the cream and a little extra broth, if
needed, to give a loose but not sloppy consistency.
* Remove from the heat and season to taste with salt and pepper. Serve
sprinkled with the parsley and extra grated Parmesan.

yummy vegetable and cashew nut burgers

Nuts contain high amounts of protein, and although children can be a little fussy about them, the flavor of the roasted nuts hidden in these burgers should tempt them. Alternatively, leave out the nuts and you still get a delicious, nutty flavor from the brown rice.

½ cup raw, unsalted cashew nuts
1 tablespoon olive oil
1 red onion, chopped
1 carrot, grated
½ small leek, carefully washed and chopped
½ cup sliced mushrooms
1 garlic clove, crushed
¼ teaspoon chopped fresh thyme leaves
¾ cup cooked brown rice (¼ cup uncooked)
1 tablespoon soy sauce
⅓ cup grated Gruyère
1 cup fresh bread crumbs
1 tablespoon honey
1 egg yolk
salt and freshly ground black pepper, to season
all-purpose flour, for dusting
2 tablespoons canola oil, for frying

* Preheat the oven to 350°F. Spread the cashew nuts on a baking sheet and roast for 8 to 10 minutes. Watch carefully, as after about 5 minutes the nuts brown quickly. Alternatively, buy roasted, unsalted cashew nuts.
* Heat the olive oil in a large frying pan with the onion, carrot, leek, mushrooms, garlic, and thyme. Sauté for 10 minutes or until the vegetables are soft and the liquid has evaporated. Add the rice and cook for 1 minute. Allow to cool slightly.
* Put the cashews in a food processor and pulse 6 or 7 times until coarsely chopped. Add the rice mixture and the soy sauce, Gruyère, bread crumbs, honey, and egg yolk with some seasoning and pulse 5 or 6 times until just combined.
* Form into 6 or 8 patties with flour-dusted hands (the mixture is a bit wet). Refrigerate for a minimum of 1 hour or overnight. Heat the canola oil in a nonstick frying pan, dust the patties with flour, and gently fry for about 3 minutes each side.

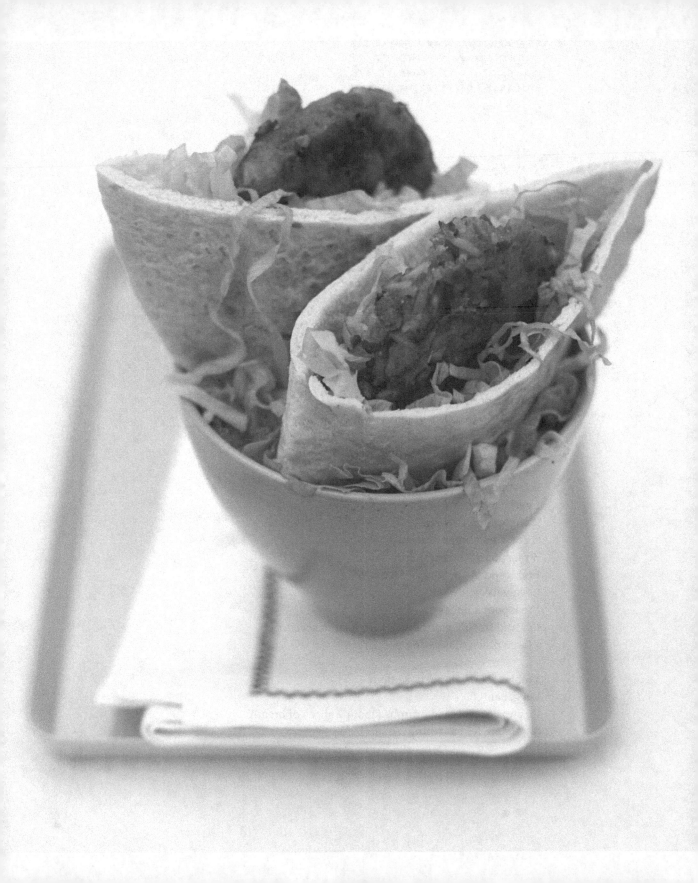

annabel's mini vegetable burgers

Getting your child to eat vegetables isn't easy, but turning veggies into a burger makes life a lot easier. Mushrooms, carrot, leek, and onion all disappear into these burgers. The soy sauce, honey, Gruyère, and cayenne pepper add to the delicious flavor. These burgers freeze very well, too, on a tray lined with plastic wrap. Once they are frozen, you can wrap each one individually so that you can remove as many as you need at any time.

1 medium potato
2 tablespoons olive oil
1 small red onion, chopped
1 medium carrot, grated
¼ leek, carefully washed and finely chopped
½ cup chopped brown mushrooms
½ teaspoon chopped fresh thyme leaves
1 garlic clove, crushed
¾ cup grated Gruyère
½ cup fresh bread crumbs
½ teaspoon Worcestershire sauce
1 tablespoon soy sauce
1 egg yolk
2 teaspoons honey
salt and freshly ground black pepper, to season
a large pinch of cayenne pepper
COATING
3 tablespoons all-purpose flour
1 egg, beaten
1½ cups fresh bread crumbs (about 2 slices of bread)
canola oil, for sautéeing

* Boil the potato, unpeeled, in lightly salted water until tender, approximately 25 minutes.
* Drain, and when cool enough to handle, peel and grate into a large bowl.
* Meanwhile, put the olive oil in a large nonstick frying pan. Sauté the onion for 3 minutes, then add the carrot, leek, mushrooms, thyme, and garlic and cook for another 10 minutes. Allow to cool slightly.
* Add the vegetables to the grated potato. Mix in the Gruyère, bread crumbs, Worcestershire sauce, soy sauce, egg yolk, and honey, and season to taste with salt, pepper, and cayenne. Form into 12 small burgers. Coat each burger with the flour, dip into the beaten egg, and then into the bread crumbs.
* In a large frying pan, heat the canola oil. Sauté as many burgers as will comfortably fit in the pan, flipping at least once, until they are golden on both sides.

focaccia pizza

Pizza tends to be popular even with fussy kids, so try adding some extra toppings such as vegetables or cooked chicken. Once these are covered by the layer of cheese, your child might be more willing to accept them.

FOR THE SAUCE
1 teaspoon olive oil
½ red onion, chopped
1 tablespoon tomato paste
2 teaspoons sun-dried tomato pesto
1 tablespoon water
salt and freshly ground black pepper, to season

one 3-inch focaccia square, split in half
2 or 3 toppings (see suggested toppings, page 44)
½ cup grated Cheddar or mozzarella

* Preheat the broiler. To make the sauce, heat the olive oil and sauté the onion for 5 minutes. Remove from the heat, stir in the tomato paste, pesto, and water, and season to taste with salt and pepper.
* Put the two halves of the focaccia on a baking sheet cut side up. Spread the sauce on top and add the toppings. Scatter the cheese on top.
* Broil the pizzas for 4 minutes or until the cheese is bubbling and golden. Transfer to plates using a spatula. Allow to cool slightly before serving.

☆ Focaccia is popular in Italy. The olive oil–enriched dough used to make the bread is similar to pizza dough and makes a tasty base for a quick pizza. If using unbaked focaccia, split it unbaked, add the toppings, and bake for 8 to 10 minutes at 400°F. Other good bases for making your own pizzas are split and toasted English muffins, or 5-inch lengths of baguette, halved.

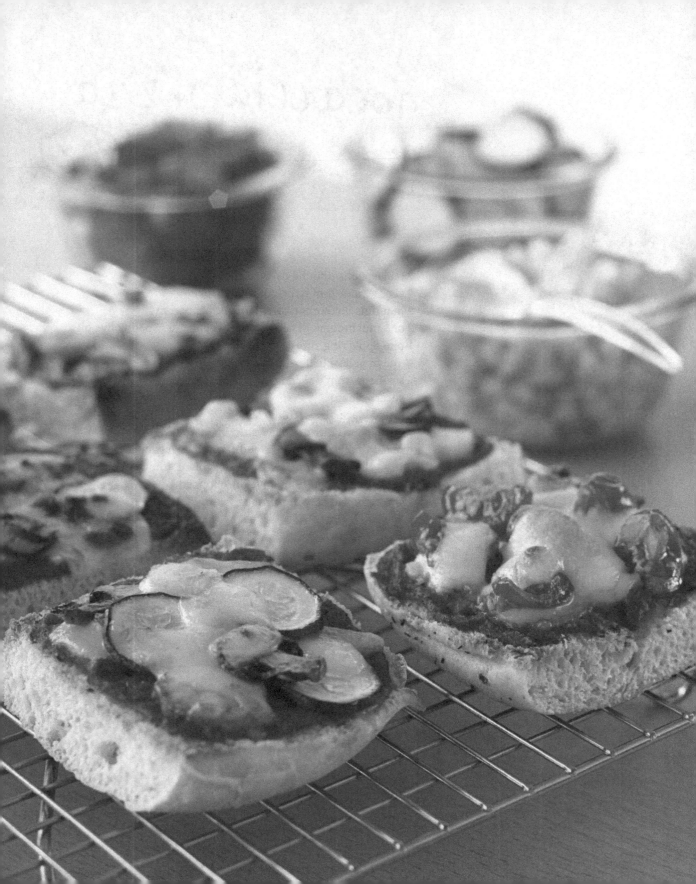

focaccia pizza

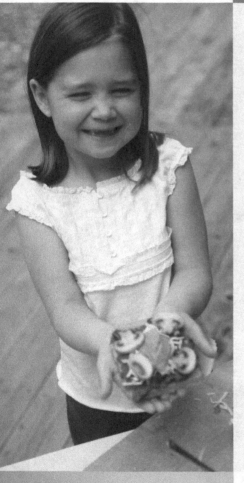

SUGGESTED TOPPINGS (ENOUGH FOR 2 PIZZAS)

2 tablespoons drained canned corn
2 slices wafer-thin ham, cut into strips
2 handfuls diced chorizo, salami, or pepperoni
2 or 3 mushrooms, sliced and sautéed in 1 teaspoon olive oil
1 pineapple ring, diced
¼ red or yellow bell pepper, diced
2 scallions, thinly sliced
4 slices tomato
4 pitted black olives, thinly sliced
2 tablespoons diced cooked chicken
roasted or stir-fried mixed Mediterranean vegetables
    (e.g., sliced zucchini, red onion, eggplant, tomato, bell pepper)
2 sun-dried tomatoes in olive oil, chopped
2 slices cooked bacon, crumbled

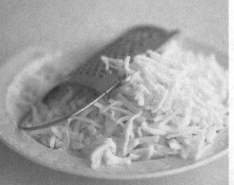

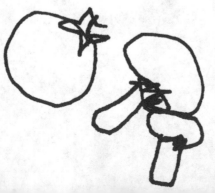

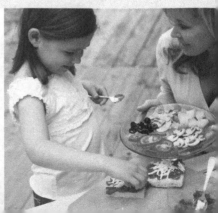

annabel's secret tomato sauce

Shh … Don't tell anyone! There are five vegetables hiding inside this super-tasty tomato sauce.

1 tablespoon olive oil
1 small red onion, chopped
½ leek, carefully washed and finely chopped
1 garlic clove, crushed
¼ red bell pepper, chopped
½ medium carrot, chopped
½ medium zucchini, chopped
one 14.5-ounce can diced tomatoes
⅔ cup vegetable broth
3 tablespoons tomato paste
1 teaspoon superfine sugar
1 tablespoon torn fresh basil leaves (optional)
salt and freshly ground black pepper, to season

* Heat the oil in a pan and sauté the onion and leek for approximately 3 minutes, stirring occasionally. Add the garlic and sauté for 1 minute. Add the bell pepper, carrot, and zucchini, and cook for another 3 minutes, stirring occasionally. Add the tomatoes, broth, tomato paste, and sugar, and stir for approximately 1 minute. Simmer uncovered for 25 to 30 minutes, stirring occasionally, until thickened. Stir in the basil leaves, if using. Transfer to a blender and blitz the sauce to a puree. Season to taste with salt and pepper.

cheesy zucchini sticks

Zucchini is sometimes challenging for younger children, as they can find its texture a little slimy. But these sticks have a crispy, crunchy texture and a delicious, cheesy flavor.

1 medium zucchini
1 egg
1 tablespoon milk
½ cup dried bread crumbs
¼ cup freshly grated Parmesan
salt and freshly ground black pepper, to season
3 tablespoons all-purpose flour
¼ cup canola oil

* Cut the zucchini in half lengthwise, then into 30 sticks roughly 2 inches long.
* Beat the egg and milk in a shallow dish with a fork to combine. Put the bread crumbs in a separate shallow dish and mix in the Parmesan plus salt and pepper to taste.
* Put the flour on a plate and toss the sticks in it in batches of 6. Dunk the floured zucchini in the egg and milk, then toss in the bread crumbs to coat. Transfer to a plate and repeat with the remaining zucchini.
* In a large frying pan, heat 2 tablespoons of the oil over medium heat and fry half of the sticks for 3 minutes on each side or until golden. Drain on paper towels and keep warm.
* Wipe out the pan with paper towels and repeat with the remaining 2 tablespoons oil and zucchini. Serve with ketchup.

frittata

This is delicious served hot or cold, and it's a good way to use up leftover cooked potato. You can sneak in some hidden veggies such as sautéed bell pepper or zucchini.

4 medium eggs
salt and freshly ground black pepper, to season
1 tablespoon olive oil
2 baby potatoes, cooked until tender and diced
1 plum tomato, seeded and diced
2 large scallions, thinly sliced
½ cup grated Cheddar

* Preheat the broiler. Put the eggs in a bowl and beat thoroughly with a fork and season with salt and pepper. In a medium frying pan, heat the oil gently for 1 to 2 minutes, then add the potatoes, tomato, scallions, and beaten egg. Cook on low heat for 12 to 15 minutes until set around the edges but still slightly wobbly in the middle.
* Sprinkle the Cheddar over the top of the frittata and broil for 2 to 3 minutes until the frittata is set and the cheese has melted. Slip onto a plate and cut into 4 to 6 wedges. It is also good served cold cut into squares.

☆ Alternatively, preheat the oven to 300°F. Oil 6 cups of a nonstick muffin pan with the olive oil. Divide the potatoes, tomato, scallions, and cheese among the muffin cups and then pour in the eggs. Bake for 17 to 20 minutes until just set in the center. Run a knife around the edge of the mini frittatas and lift out to serve.

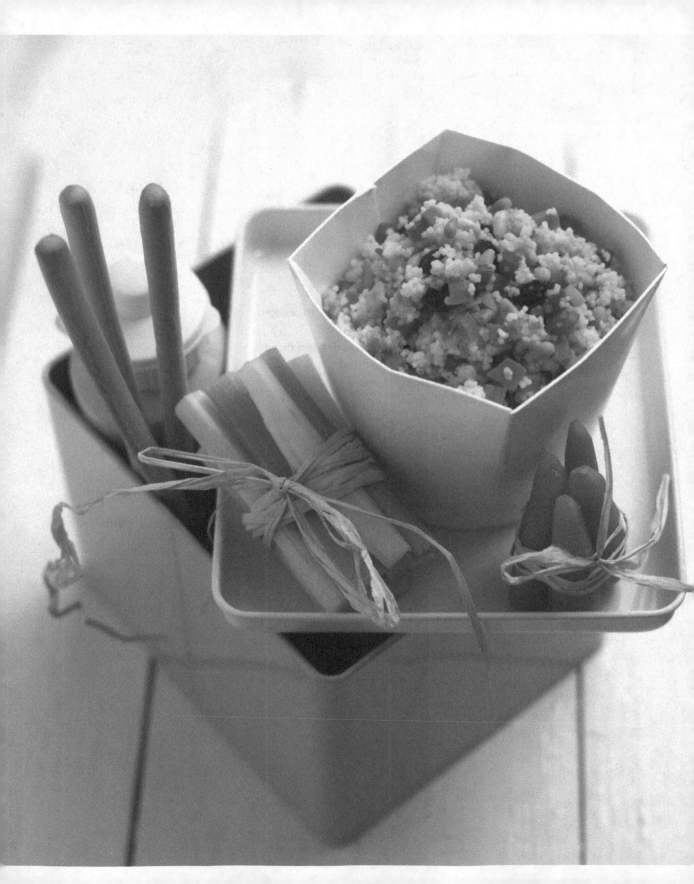

confetti couscous salad

Toast the pine nuts by frying them in a dry frying pan until golden, stirring frequently to make sure that they don't burn.

¼ cup couscous
½ cup hot vegetable broth
¼ red bell pepper, diced
¼ orange or yellow bell pepper, diced
1 small tomato, seeded and chopped
2 scallions, sliced
1 tablespoon raisins
1½ tablespoons pine nuts, toasted
salt and freshly ground black pepper, to season

DRESSING

1 tablespoon olive oil
1 teaspoon balsamic vinegar
½ teaspoon honey

* Put the couscous in a bowl. Add the hot vegetable broth, cover, and let stand for 10 minutes, then fluff up with a fork. Stir in the vegetables, raisins, and pine nuts.

* Whisk together the ingredients for the dressing and stir into the couscous. Season to taste.

☆ Couscous is grainlike pasta made from wheat, popular in Middle Eastern cuisine. You can find it in most supermarkets next to the rice section. What is really good about couscous is that it is so quick and easy to prepare. This could be an option for your child's lunch box instead of sandwiches. It's also good to keep healthy salads like this in the fridge for your child to snack on during the day.

vegetable quesadillas

A quesadilla (pronounced ke-sah-*dee*-uh) is a Tex-Mex dish that involves cooking ingredients inside tortillas. I find children like eating tortillas—one of the reasons is that they can eat them with their fingers. You can add other ingredients to this, such as some shredded cooked chicken (see page 128 for Yummy Chicken Quesadillas). To serve, you can use a store-bought salsa or guacamole or make your own.

½ red bell pepper, thinly sliced
½ yellow bell pepper, thinly sliced
1 small red onion, thinly sliced
1 garlic clove, crushed
1 tablespoon olive oil
salt and freshly ground black pepper,
   to season
a pinch of cayenne pepper (optional)

SALSA
2 medium tomatoes, seeded and diced
1 large scallion, finely chopped
½ teaspoon chopped fresh cilantro
1 teaspoon fresh lime juice
a pinch of sugar

salt and freshly ground black pepper,
   to season

GUACAMOLE
1 large avocado
1½ teaspoons fresh lemon juice
2 tablespoons cream cheese
1 to 2 tablespoons sliced scallion
1 to 2 tablespoons diced bell pepper
salt and freshly ground black pepper,
   to season

two 7-inch flour tortillas
¾ cup grated Cheddar
2 tablespoons sour cream, to serve

* Put the peppers, onion, garlic, and olive oil in a large nonstick frying pan and stir-fry for 6 to 7 minutes until the vegetables are soft. Season with salt and pepper plus cayenne pepper, if using. Set aside in a bowl.
* To make the salsa, simply mix together all the ingredients. To make the guacamole, cut the avocado in half, remove the pit, and scoop out the flesh. Mash together with the remaining ingredients.
* Wipe the frying pan with paper towels; lay a tortilla in the bottom. Spread it with the peppers and onion and sprinkle the cheese on top. Place the other tortilla on top and put the pan over medium heat. Cook for 1½ to 2 minutes until starting to brown on the bottom. Flip onto a plate and slide back into the pan to cook the other side for 1½ to 2 minutes. (If you are worried about flipping the tortillas, then brown the top for 1 to 2 minutes under a hot broiler.)
* Slide out of the pan (use a spatula to help) and cut into 6 wedges. Serve with sour cream, salsa, and guacamole.

i don't like...

avocado

(you must be joking)

cannelloni

If your child isn't keen on eating vegetables, try hiding them inside
a cannelloni. The recipe given here makes 12 to 14 crepes, which is
more than you will need for the cannelloni. However, the extra crepes
will keep in the fridge for a couple of days or can be frozen.

CREPES
1 cup all-purpose flour
a generous pinch of salt
1 large egg
1¼ cups milk
1 tablespoon butter, melted and cooled, plus extra for frying

SAUCE
Annabel's Secret Tomato Sauce (page 45)

FILLING
3 cups fresh spinach, carefully washed, or one 10-ounce package frozen
   spinach, thawed
salt
¾ cup ricotta
6 ounces diced fresh mozzarella
½ cup freshly grated Parmesan
1 egg yolk, lightly beaten
a pinch of nutmeg (optional)
freshly gound black pepper, to season

TOPPING
¼ cup diced fresh mozzarella
2 tablespoons freshly grated Parmesan

* Put the flour in a large bowl with the salt. Make a well and crack the egg into
the middle, then add ¼ cup of the milk and the melted butter and whisk to
make a thick batter. While whisking, gradually pour in the remaining 1 cup milk.
Continue pouring and whisking until you have a batter that is the consistency
of slightly thick cream. Alternatively, you can blitz all the ingredients in a
blender; transfer the batter to a bowl. Traditionally, people would say to leave

the batter for 30 minutes to allow the starch in the flour to swell, but there's no need to do this.

* Heat a heavy 8-inch frying pan over medium heat, then grease with a knob of butter. Ladle some batter (approximately 3 tablespoons) into the pan, swirling to coat the bottom of the pan. Cook for 1 to 2 minutes until golden on the bottom. Flip over, cook for another minute, then transfer the crepe to a plate. Repeat until all the batter is used. (If you are making the crepes in advance, layer them with sheets of baking parchment, cover with plastic wrap, and place in the freezer. To serve, remove from the freezer and defrost, then either microwave for a few seconds or heat in a pan with a little butter.)

* Preheat the oven to 400°F. Prepare Annabel's Secret Tomato Sauce.

* To make the filling, put the spinach into a large pan, sprinkle with salt, and cook for about 3 minutes or until the leaves have wilted. Transfer the spinach to a colander and press out the excess liquid. Place on a cutting board and chop into small pieces.

* In a bowl, mix the chopped spinach with the ricotta, mozzarella, Parmesan, egg yolk, and nutmeg, if using. Season with a little salt and pepper.

* Divide the spinach mixture among 8 crepes (roughly a heaping tablespoon each), spooning into the center of the crepe and spreading out slightly into a sausage shape. Put one of the crepes in front of you with the filling vertical. Fold in the left- and right-hand sides of the crepe, so that you have a rectangle shape, and roll up from the short edge closest to you to make a parcel. Put in an oiled baking dish seam side down and repeat with the remaining crepes.

* Pour the sauce over the cannelloni, sprinkle with the mozzarella and Parmesan, and bake for 30 minutes or until piping hot. You can also brown the top under the broiler if you like.

vegetable kebabs

Children like eating food off a stick or skewer. Here I've marinated some vegetables in balsamic vinegar and honey to give them a delicious flavor. These would be good served with chicken or beef skewers.

MARINADE

2 tablespoons olive oil
2 teaspoons balsamic vinegar
2 teaspoons honey
salt and freshly ground black pepper,
  to season

4 bamboo skewers, soaked in water for
  20 minutes
¼ yellow bell pepper, cut into big chunks
¼ orange or red bell pepper, cut into
  big chunks
1 medium zucchini, cut into ½-inch-
  thick rounds

* Combine the marinade ingredients, then soak the vegetables in this mixture for 1 to 2 hours.
* Preheat the broiler. Thread the vegetables onto the skewers and cook for 2 minutes under the broiler. Baste and cook for another 2 minutes. Turn, baste, and cook for 2 minutes, then baste and cook for 1 minute more.

hawaiian chicken salad

Most children love sweet, juicy pineapple and so should be tempted by this salad. It would make a good alternative to sandwiches in your child's lunch box.

scant ½ cup long-grain white rice
3 large scallions, sliced
¼ cup cubed cooked chicken
¼ cup thawed frozen peas
3 tablespoons drained canned corn
half an 8-ounce can pineapple pieces in
  juice, drained, reserving 2 tablespoons
  juice for the dressing
1 tomato, seeded and diced

DRESSING

2 tablespoons canola oil
2 tablespoons pineapple juice (reserved
  from can)
1 teaspoon fresh lemon juice
salt and freshly ground black pepper,
  to season

* Cook the rice according to the package directions and leave to cool. Mix together with the remaining ingredients for the chicken salad. Whisk together all the ingredients for the dressing and toss with the salad.

orzo salad

Orzo is tiny pasta that looks like grains of rice. If you can't find it, then use tiny shell-shaped pasta instead.

⅓ cup orzo
2 tablespoons peas, cooked from frozen
¼ cup drained canned corn
½ cup cubed cooked chicken

DRESSING
1 tablespoon mayonnaise
1 tablespoon sour cream or Greek-style
   yogurt
1 teaspoon water
½ teaspoon white wine vinegar
1½ teaspoons snipped fresh chives

* Cook the orzo according to the package directions. Drain and mix with the peas, corn, and cooked chicken.
* Whisk together all the ingredients for the dressing and toss with the salad.

carrot and cucumber salad

Most kids love cucumber, so here I've combined it with carrot, which is a lot more nutritious, as it's a great source of beta-carotene. The Japanese make this salad using seaweed and cucumber, and it's delicious. However, seaweed is pretty hard to find, so I have used carrot, cucumber, and bean sprouts instead.

1 large carrot
½ cucumber, preferably English or
   hothouse
½ cup bean sprouts

DRESSING
1 tablespoon soy sauce
1 tablespoon rice wine vinegar
1 tablespoon canola oil
1 tablespoon honey
1 teaspoon mirin
1 teaspoon Asian sesame oil

1 tablespoon sesame seeds, toasted
   (optional), for sprinkling

* Peel the carrot and cucumber, then use a swivel peeler to peel off thin strips. Combine with the bean sprouts.
* Whisk together all the ingredients for the dressing, pour onto the vegetables, and toss. Sprinkle with the sesame seeds, if using.

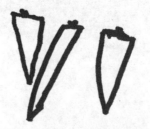

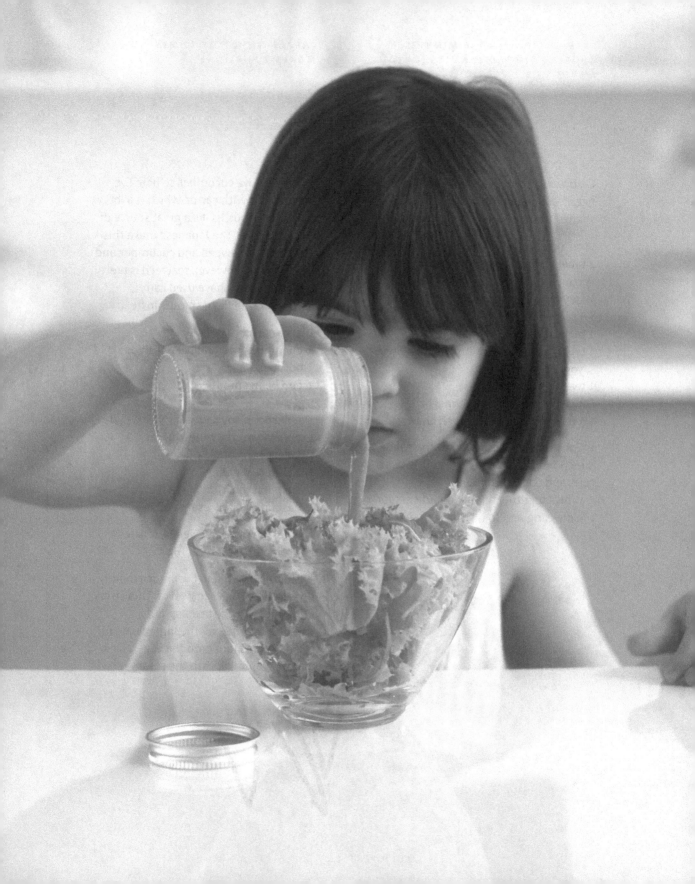

favorite salad dressings

The secret to getting your child to enjoy eating salad is to find a dressing that he or she really likes. I made up a Japanese-style dressing called Dressing for Dinner in my *Favorite Family Meals* cookbook, which my children absolutely love. I make up six large bottles at a time, as they can't get enough of it, and use it not only as a dressing but also as a dip for vegetables and as a sauce on foods such as rice or chicken. Try out these tasty dressings and see if you can find one that your child really enjoys.

creamy caesar dressing

This is an easy version of the popular salad dressing.

¼ cup mayonnaise
2 tablespoons freshly grated Parmesan
¼ teaspoon fresh lemon juice
3 or 4 drops Worcestershire sauce (to taste)
¼ cup cold milk
1 small garlic clove, crushed
salt and freshly ground black pepper,
   to season

* Whisk together all the ingredients. Store in a jar in the fridge for up to 2 weeks and shake well before serving.

tomato balsamic dressing

This is a particular favorite of mine. If your balsamic vinegar is very sharp, then you might like to add an extra pinch of sugar—it's worth spending a little extra to get a mature balsamic vinegar with a more rounded, sweeter flavor.

2 large ripe tomatoes, roughly chopped
6 tablespoons olive oil
3 tablespoons balsamic vinegar
2 teaspoons tomato paste
4 sun-dried tomatoes in olive oil,
    chopped
1 tablespoon sugar (optional)
salt and freshly ground black pepper,
    to season

* Put all of the ingredients into a blender and whiz for 2 minutes, until thoroughly pureed. Strain the dressing. Store in a jar in the fridge for up to 2 weeks and shake well before serving.

herby ranch dressing

Traditionally, ranch dressing is made with buttermilk, but I prefer to use thick Greek-style yogurt and fresh lemon juice. This also makes a nice dip for vegetable sticks—just reduce the water to 2 tablespoons.

3 tablespoons mayonnaise
3 tablespoons Greek-style yogurt
1 tablespoon fresh lemon juice
¼ cup cold water
½ small garlic clove, crushed (optional)
2 teaspoons snipped fresh chives
1 teaspoon chopped fresh parsley
1 teaspoon chopped fresh cilantro, dill,
    or mint
salt and freshly ground black pepper,
    to season

* Whisk together all the ingredients. Store in a jar in the fridge for up to 2 weeks and shake well before serving.

oriental salad

I find that children really like the texture of fried rice noodles, so I've combined them with some super-nutritious ingredients such as sunflower and pumpkin seeds, napa cabbage, and snow peas and tossed everything in a divine dressing. It's so good that I often serve this to friends who come over for supper. Everyone always asks me for the recipe.

canola or peanut oil, for deep-frying
a few cubes of stale bread
2 ounces (about 2 handfuls) thin rice noodles
3 tablespoons sunflower seeds
3 tablespoons pumpkin seeds
¼ head napa cabbage, shredded
2 handfuls snow peas, cut into matchsticks
2 handfuls bean sprouts

DRESSING
¼ cup canola oil
3 tablespoons honey
2 tablespoons red wine vinegar
1 tablespoon soy sauce
1 teaspoon Asian sesame oil
salt and freshly ground black pepper, to season

* Preheat the oven to 400°F. Put 2 inches oil in a large, deep pan over medium heat until a cube of bread dropped into the oil turns golden brown in 30 seconds. Pull the noodles apart. Drop a small handful of them into the hot oil (be careful, as they may spit a bit). The noodles will puff up almost at once, so remove them immediately with a slotted spoon and drain on a tray lined with a double layer of paper towels. Allow the oil to reheat for a minute before frying the next batch.
* Spread the seeds on a baking sheet and toast for 8 to 10 minutes, stirring halfway through. Watch carefully after the first 5 minutes, as they can burn easily. Allow to cool.
* Mix the cabbage, snow peas, and bean sprouts with the noodles and seeds in a big bowl. Whisk together all the ingredients for the dressing, pour onto the salad, and toss.

vegetable chips

I don't normally like beets or parsnips, but when they are cooked this way, I can't get enough of them. These make a good alternative to a bag of potato chips.

8 ounces mixed root vegetables (such as sweet potatoes, parsnips, carrots, and beets)
canola oil, for deep-frying
a few cubes of stale bread
sea salt and freshly ground black pepper, to season

* Peel the vegetables and slice them wafer thin using a vegetable peeler or mandoline slicer. Rinse and dry the slices.
* Put enough oil in a deep-fat fryer or large pan to come one-third to halfway up the sides. Heat the oil and test whether it is hot enough by tossing a bread cube into the pan. If it turns golden within about 30 seconds, the oil is ready. Add the vegetables separately and fry in batches. They will turn golden within a few minutes. Remove them at once using the basket of the deep-fryer or a slotted spoon and drain on paper towels. Sprinkle with salt and pepper. Allow to cool and then store in an airtight container.

☆ You can also cook the chips in the oven. Simply toss in a large bowl with some oil and seasoning, spread out on a nonstick baking sheet, and bake at 400°F for 12 to 15 minutes until golden, turning halfway through.

PREPARATION TIME 10 MINUTES
COOKING TIME 30 MINUTES
MAKES 3 PORTIONS

PREPARATION TIME 10 MINUTES
COOKING TIME 30 MINUTES
MAKES 3 OR 4 PORTIONS

spicy potato wedges

If your child likes French fries, you might
want to opt for a healthier version that is
baked in the oven rather than fried. These
are particularly good when dipped in sour
cream or Herby Ranch Dressing (page 58).

2 medium white potatoes (such as
    Yukon Gold), well scrubbed
2 tablespoons canola oil
1 to 2 teaspoons fajita spice mix
salt, to season

* Preheat the oven to 400°F.
* Cut the potatoes in half lengthwise,
then cut each half into 6 wedges. Put in a
colander and rinse well with cold water. Pat
dry thoroughly with a clean kitchen towel
or paper towels.
* Put the oil and spice mix in a large bowl
and mix. Toss the wedges in the oil and lay
out on a large baking sheet (you can line
the baking sheet with foil for an easy
cleanup). Bake for 30 minutes, turning
halfway through. Allow to cool for
5 minutes, then sprinkle with a little
salt before serving.

☆ Mix a little salt and pepper with paprika,
garlic powder, or rosemary as an alternative
flavoring for the wedges.

root vegetable oven fries

Another delicious alternative to ordinary
French fries. This might be a good way
to encourage your child to try other
vegetables. You could brush the vegetables
with a little honey for the last 5 to 10
minutes (not earlier, or it will burn),
and you could season with a little ground
coriander if your child likes this.

1 medium parsnip
1 small sweet potato
1 large carrot
2 tablespoons canola oil
salt, to season

* Preheat the oven to 400°F.
* Peel the vegetables and cut into sticks
roughly 2 to 3 inches long and ½ inch thick.
Put in a large bowl with the oil and toss to
coat thoroughly.
* Spread out on a large baking sheet
(lined with foil if you want to make the
cleanup easier) and bake for 30 minutes,
turning halfway through. Allow to cool for
5 minutes, then sprinkle with a little salt
before serving.

mini corn fritters

My daughter Lara really likes these. She often has them as a snack, so I keep a supply of them in the freezer. To freeze them, wrap the cooled fritters in foil in a single layer with 2 fritters per package. To serve, preheat the oven to 350°F and put the frozen fritters on a baking sheet. Bake for approximately 8 minutes until hot. These fritters can also be made with gluten-free flour.

¼ cup all-purpose flour
½ teaspoon baking powder
¼ teaspoon salt
1 large egg
1 cup drained canned corn
1 large or 2 small scallions, thinly sliced
2 tablespoons canola oil, for frying

* Whiz together all the ingredients except the oil in a food processor for 1 minute to make a batter.
* Heat a little of the oil in a large frying pan and drop in tablespoonfuls of the batter. Cook for 1 to 1½ minutes in two batches of 5 until golden on the undersides, then carefully turn and cook for another minute. You can use the back of a spoon to help push the fritter onto a spatula to make turning easier. Drain briefly on paper towels before serving.

mini
corn fritters

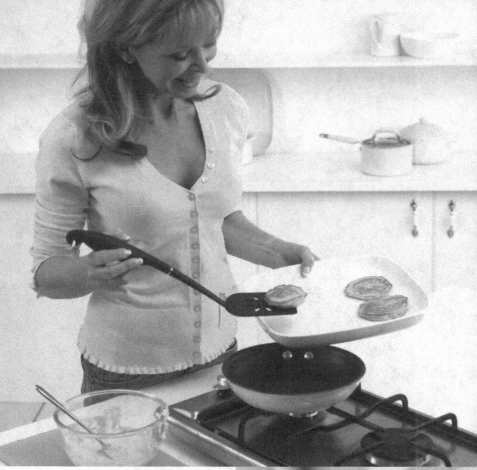

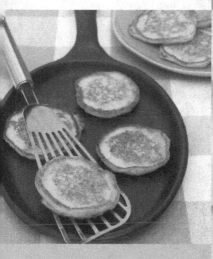

TIP
Experts recommend that we eat 5 daily servings of fruit and vegetables. Three tablespoons of corn counts as one serving of fruit and vegetables.

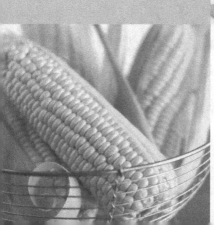

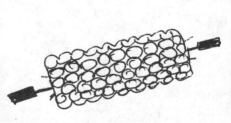

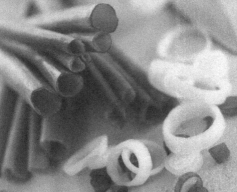

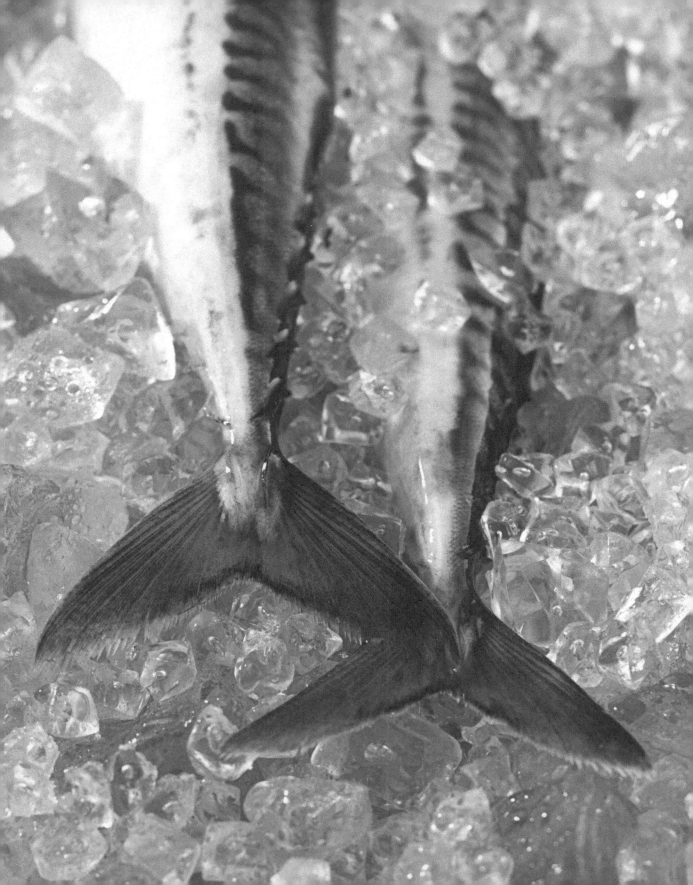

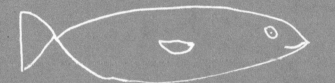

funky fish

top tips

how to get your child to eat fish

* There's nothing worse than dry, overcooked fish. Raw fish is slightly translucent. As soon as it becomes opaque all the way through, it is cooked.

* Always check carefully for bones. Even filleted fish can have small bones, and this could put your child off eating fish.

* There are lots of tasty ways to coat fish: try using crushed cornflakes, popcorn and grated cheese, or even crushed crackers.

* Children like to eat with their fingers, so fix recipes like marinated salmon on a skewer, mini fish cakes, or shrimp toast.

* Sardines mashed with a little ketchup, or tuna mixed with corn, scallion, and mayonnaise make a good sandwich filling.

* Make individual fish pies in mini ramekins. It looks much more appealing than a dollop of fish pie on a plate, and you can make a few at a time and pop some in the freezer.

* Children can be fascinated by the different kinds of fish in a fish store. You might like to take them with you occasionally and see if they can name the different types of fish.

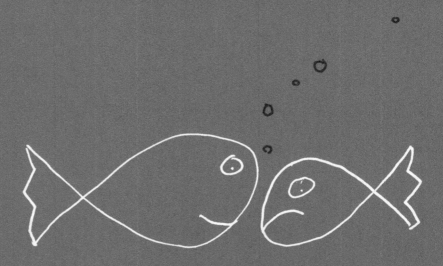

super salmon wrap

Unlike canned tuna, a can of salmon contains some brain-boosting omega-3 fatty acids.

1 tablespoon mayonnaise
1½ tablespoons ketchup
2 drops Tabasco sauce
½ teaspoon fresh lemon juice
2 tablespoons canned red salmon, flaked
½ tomato, seeded and diced
1½-inch-thick piece cucumber, diced
1 small scallion, thinly sliced
one 7-inch flour tortilla

* Mix together the mayonnaise, ketchup, Tabasco, and lemon juice. Stir in the flaked salmon, tomato, cucumber, and scallion.
* Heat the tortilla for 20 seconds on full power in the microwave, or for about 15 seconds in a dry frying pan. Arrange the filling near one edge of the tortilla and roll up. Cut the tortilla in half diagonally and serve.

annabel's tasty shrimp wrap

Wraps are the new, trendy sandwich, and shrimp in cocktail sauce are generally popular with children, so this makes a good combination. As you can see, it's very easy to make your own cocktail sauce. This would also make a good sandwich filling.

2 tablespoons mayonnaise
1 teaspoon ketchup
½ teaspoon fresh lemon juice
2 or 3 drops Worcestershire sauce
½ cup cooked peeled small shrimp
½ medium tomato, seeded and diced
1 small scallion, thinly sliced
one 7-inch flour tortilla
a handful of shredded lettuce

* Mix together the mayonnaise, ketchup, lemon juice, and Worcestershire sauce. Stir in the shrimp, tomato, and scallion.
* Heat the tortilla for 20 seconds on full power in a microwave, or for about 15 seconds in a dry frying pan. Arrange the shrimp mixture near one edge of the tortilla, cover with the shredded lettuce, and roll up. Cut the tortilla in half diagonally and serve.

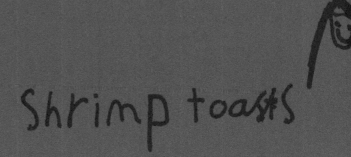

shrimp toasts

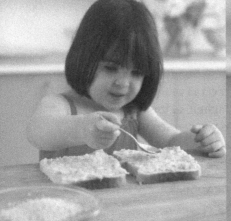

TIP
When I take my children to a Chinese restaurant, they love the food, so it's a good idea to make your own Chinese food at home and get your child to help in the kitchen.

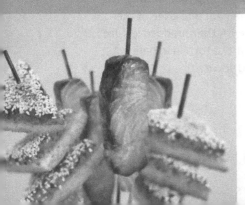

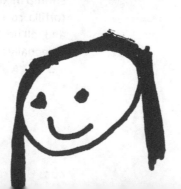

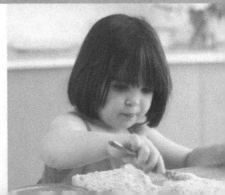

shrimp toasts

Ever notice how much kids eat when you take them out for a Chinese meal? So why don't they eat like that at home?! Shrimp toasts are always popular, and there's usually a fight over who is going to eat the last one. So maybe here's a way to get your child to appreciate your home cooking.

⅔ cup cooked peeled small shrimp
1 medium egg white
1 large scallion, thinly sliced
a large pinch of salt
2 slices white bread, crusts removed
1 tablespoon sesame seeds
¼ cup canola oil, for frying

* Put the shrimp, egg white, and scallion into a food processor with the salt and whiz to a paste. Spread the mixture over the 2 slices of bread. Sprinkle the sesame seeds on top and cut each slice into 4 squares or triangles.
* Heat 3 tablespoons of the oil in a large nonstick frying pan over medium heat for 2 to 3 minutes. Fry the toasts bread side down for 2½ to 3 minutes until golden on the undersides. Reduce the heat slightly. Turn the toasts over, add the remaining 1 tablespoon oil, and fry for another 2 to 3 minutes until golden. Transfer the cooked toasts (bread side down) to a double layer of paper towels and allow to cool for a couple of minutes before serving.

salmon on a stick with stir-fried noodles

These salmon "lollipops" with a slightly sweet glaze are a good way to tempt children who may shy away from fish.

2 tablespoons fresh orange juice

1½ tablespoons honey

2 teaspoons soy sauce

6 ounces skinless salmon fillet (needs to be 1 inch thick, so not tail end)

2 bamboo skewers, soaked in water for 20 minutes

NOODLES

3 ounces Chinese-stye dried thin egg noodles (lo mein), cooked
   according to package directions and drained, or cooked
   thin bean thread (cellophane) noodles

½ teaspoon Asian sesame oil

1 teaspoon canola oil

a handful of snow peas, cut into matchsticks

¼ red or orange bell pepper, cut into thin strips

2 scallions, sliced

a handful of bean sprouts

1 tablespoon soy sauce

1 tablespoon sesame seeds, lightly toasted

* Put the orange juice, honey, and soy sauce in a small pan. Bring to a boil and cook for about 1 minute or until thickened slightly. Allow to cool.
* Preheat the broiler. Meanwhile, cut the salmon in half lengthwise and thread onto the skewers. Fold any thin belly pieces over so that the fish is even in thickness. Put on a foil-lined broiler tray. Brush on some sauce and broil for 2 minutes. Brush again and broil for 1 minute. Turn the salmon over, and repeat. Reserve any leftover sauce.
* If the salmon is particularly thick, baste the sides with the juices from the pan and broil for 1 minute each side (as close to the broiler as possible). Keep the salmon warm while you prepare the noodles.
* Toss the noodles in the sesame oil. Heat the canola oil in a wok and stir-fry the snow peas, pepper, and scallions for 2 to 3 minutes. Add the bean sprouts and noodles and cook for 1½ to 2 minutes. Bring the sauce to a boil; toss the noodles with the sauce and 2 tablespoons water, the soy sauce, and sesame seeds.

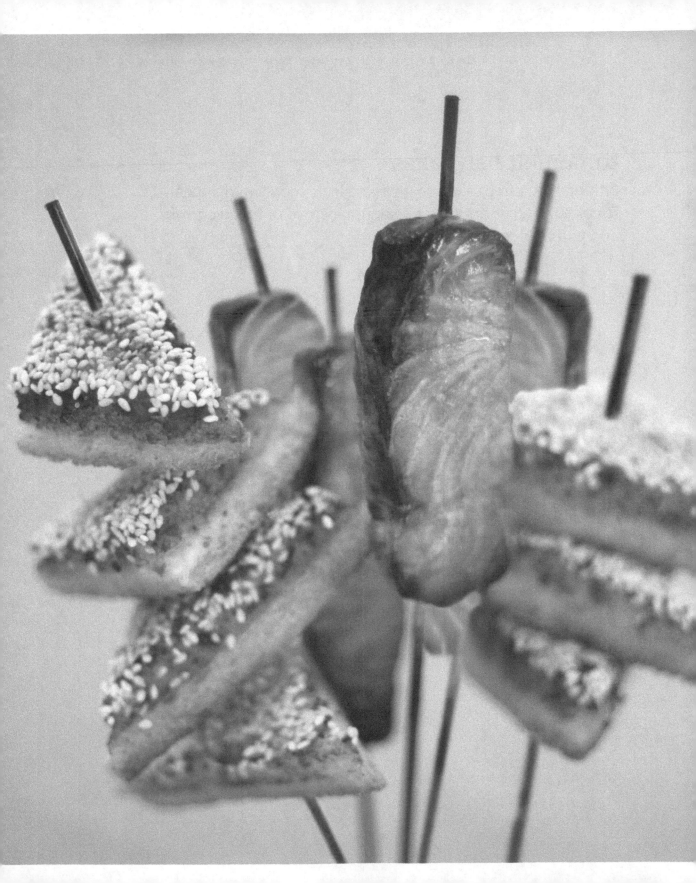

tuna melt fish cakes

Adding ketchup to a recipe gives it a little more child appeal.
For a gluten-free option, use polenta instead of bread crumbs
and gluten-free flour for dusting.

2 medium potatoes
2 tablespoons mayonnaise
2 tablespoons ketchup
two 6-ounce cans tuna in water, drained and flaked
4 scallions, finely chopped
1 teaspoon fresh lemon juice
3 tablespoons all-purpose flour, seasoned with salt and pepper, for dusting
1 egg, beaten with 1 tablespoon milk
⅔ cup dried bread crumbs
¾ cup grated Cheddar

* Peel and boil the potatoes in lightly salted water until soft, drain, and mash
with the mayonnaise and ketchup. Stir in the tuna, scallions, and lemon juice.
* Preheat the oven to 400°F.
* Form 8 fish cakes. Dust the cakes with the flour, dip in the beaten egg and
milk, and coat in the bread crumbs.
* Put the fish cakes on an oiled baking sheet and bake for 10 minutes. Turn over
and bake for another 5 minutes, then sprinkle the grated Cheddar on top and
bake for 5 minutes more. (You can brown them under the broiler for a couple
of minutes after baking if you like.)

salmon fish cakes

There are two versions of these salmon fish cakes. You can make them without a bread crumb coating (as here), or if you want them as child-friendly finger food, roll the mixture into 12 balls, dust in flour, dip in beaten egg, then coat in bread crumbs. You will need about ½ cup fresh white bread crumbs. You can then either shallow-fry or cook in a deep-fryer.

1 medium potato
3 ounces skinless salmon fillet
a squeeze of lemon juice (for microwave method)
a knob of butter (for microwave method)
½ cup fish broth (for poaching)
2 scallions, chopped
1 teaspoon chili sauce
2 tablespoons ketchup
1½ teaspoons mayonnaise
salt and freshly ground black pepper, to season
1 tablespoon all-purpose flour, seasoned with salt and pepper, for dusting
2 tablespoons canola oil, for frying

* Boil the unpeeled potato in lightly salted water for 25 to 30 minutes until tender when pierced with a table knife. Drain, and when cool enough to handle, peel and mash. Cook the salmon, covered, in the microwave for a couple of minutes with the lemon juice and butter. Allow to cool slightly, then flake. Alternatively, poach for a couple of minutes in the fish broth. Drain if poaching, and flake onto a plate.
* Mix the potato with the scallions, chili sauce, ketchup, mayonnaise, and salt and pepper to taste. Fold in the flaked salmon, being careful not to break up the fish too much. Take tablespoonfuls of the mixture and form into small cakes. Dust with the seasoned flour.
* Heat the oil in a nonstick pan and fry the fish cakes for 2 to 3 minutes on each side until golden.

PREPARATION TIME 5 MINUTES
COOKING TIME 15 MINUTES
MAKES 2 PORTIONS

salmon and cod in a chive sauce

That old saying "fish is good for the brain" is absolutely true. Oil-rich fish such as salmon, fresh tuna, and sardines are a good source of brain-boosting omega-3 fatty acids, which are vital for brain function and can help the performance of dyslexic and hyperactive children.

1 large shallot, diced
1 tablespoon butter
2 tablespoons white wine vinegar
1 tablespoon all-purpose flour
1 cup fish broth
3 tablespoons heavy cream
½ teaspoon fresh lemon juice
2 teaspoons finely snipped fresh chives
4 ounces skinless salmon fillet, cut into 1-inch cubes
4 ounces skinless cod fillet, cut into 1-inch cubes
¼ to ⅓ cup frozen peas

* Cook the shallot in the butter over low heat for about 5 minutes until soft but not colored. Add the vinegar and boil until just evaporated. Stir in the flour and cook gently for 2 minutes, stirring occasionally.
* Whisk in the broth. Bring to a boil, stirring, and boil until reduced by half. Remove from the heat and stir in the cream, lemon juice, and chives.
* Put the fish in a suitable microwave dish together with the peas. Add the sauce. Cover with plastic wrap, prick the top, and cook in the microwave at full power for about 2½ minutes. Alternatively, add the fish to the saucepan with the peas and poach in the sauce for about 4 minutes until cooked through. Serve with fluffy white rice if you like.

fabulous fish pie

1 pound potatoes, peeled and cut into chunks
2 medium carrots, sliced
3 tablespoons milk
4 tablespoons (½ stick) butter
salt and white pepper, to season
4 cups fresh baby spinach, carefully washed

WHITE SAUCE
2 tablespoons butter
1 small onion, chopped
¼ cup all-purpose flour
½ cup milk
½ cup chicken or vegetable broth
¼ teaspoon Dijon mustard

9 ounces skinless salmon fillet, cut into 1-inch cubes
9 ounces skinless cod fillet, cut into 1-inch cubes
1 tablespoon finely chopped fresh parsley
1 bay leaf
½ cup grated sharp Cheddar
salt and white pepper, to season
1 egg, lightly beaten

* Bring a pan of lightly salted water to a boil, add the potatoes, reduce the heat, and cook for 15 minutes. Steam the carrots for about 20 minutes until tender. Combine the vegetables and mash with the milk and half the butter until smooth. Season to taste.

* Place the spinach in a hot pan for a few minutes until wilted. Drain and gently squeeze out the excess water. Melt the remaining butter in the pan, sauté the spinach for a couple of minutes, and season.

* Preheat the oven to 350°F. Melt the butter and sauté the onion until softened. Add the flour and cook for about 30 seconds, stirring occasionally. Gradually stir in the milk, broth, and mustard. Bring to a boil and cook for a few minutes. Add the fish, parsley, and bay leaf and simmer for 4 to 5 minutes. Remove the bay leaf and stir in the cheese until melted. Season well.

* Put the fish with the sauce into a 7-inch round ovenproof dish. Arrange the spinach on top, then cover with the mashed potato. Make a design with fork tines and brush with the beaten egg. Bake for 30 to 35 minutes.

mini fish pies

I design the menus for one of the largest chains of day care centers in the UK, and one of the children's favorite dishes is this fish pie. Another is my fruity curried chicken, so it's interesting to see that children often have more sophisticated taste than we imagine. Making food look attractive is important, and so it seems much more appealing to serve an individual fish pie rather than a dollop of food on the plate.

POTATO TOPPING

1¾ pounds potatoes, peeled and cut into chunks
2 tablespoons butter
½ cup milk
¼ cup freshly grated Parmesan
salt and freshly ground black pepper, to season

SAUCE

3 tablespoons butter
1 large shallot, diced
2 tablespoons white wine vinegar
¼ cup all-purpose flour
2 cups fish broth
⅔ cup heavy cream
1½ teaspoons chopped fresh dill or snipped fresh chives
salt and freshly ground black pepper, to season

SALMON AND COD FILLING

9 ounces skinless salmon fillet, cut into ¾-inch pieces
9 ounces skinless cod fillet, cut into ¾-inch pieces
¾ cup cooked peeled small shrimp
½ cup frozen peas

1 egg, lightly beaten

* Boil the potatoes in lightly salted water. Drain and mash with the butter, milk, and Parmesan and season to taste.
* To make the sauce, melt the butter and sauté the shallot for 5 to 6 minutes until soft. Add the white wine vinegar and boil for 2 to 3 minutes until the liquid has evaporated. Stir in the flour to make a roux. Gradually, stir in the fish broth and then cook over medium heat, stirring continuously. Bring to a boil, then cook, stirring, until thickened. Remove from the heat and stir in the cream and the chopped dill or chives. Season well, as the fish is unseasoned.
* Preheat the oven to 400°F.
* Divide the fish, shrimp, and peas among 4 to 6 mini ramekins (depending on the size) and add the sauce. If you have time, allow the filling to cool and become less liquid and easier to cover with the mashed potato without the potato sinking into the filling. Brush the potato topping with a little beaten egg. Bake for 25 minutes.

sizzling asian shrimp

A lot of my more popular recipes for children are Asian-style dishes. It's also good to flavor thin fillets of white fish with garlic, ginger, scallion, and soy sauce and cook them wrapped in foil.

2 teaspoons canola oil
1 teaspoon grated fresh ginger
1 garlic clove, crushed
¾ pound peeled raw large shrimp, or frozen shrimp, thawed
2 teaspoons Asian sesame oil
2 large or 4 small scallions, thinly sliced
1 tablespoon fresh lime juice
a handful of fresh cilantro leaves, to serve (optional)

* Heat the canola oil in a wok or skillet until sizzling. Add the ginger, garlic, and shrimp and cook for 1 to 1½ minutes, then turn the shrimp over and cook for another 1 to 2 minutes, until the shrimp have turned pink. Add the sesame oil, scallions, and lime juice and stir for 30 seconds or until fragrant.
* Remove from the heat and serve with the cilantro leaves scattered on top.

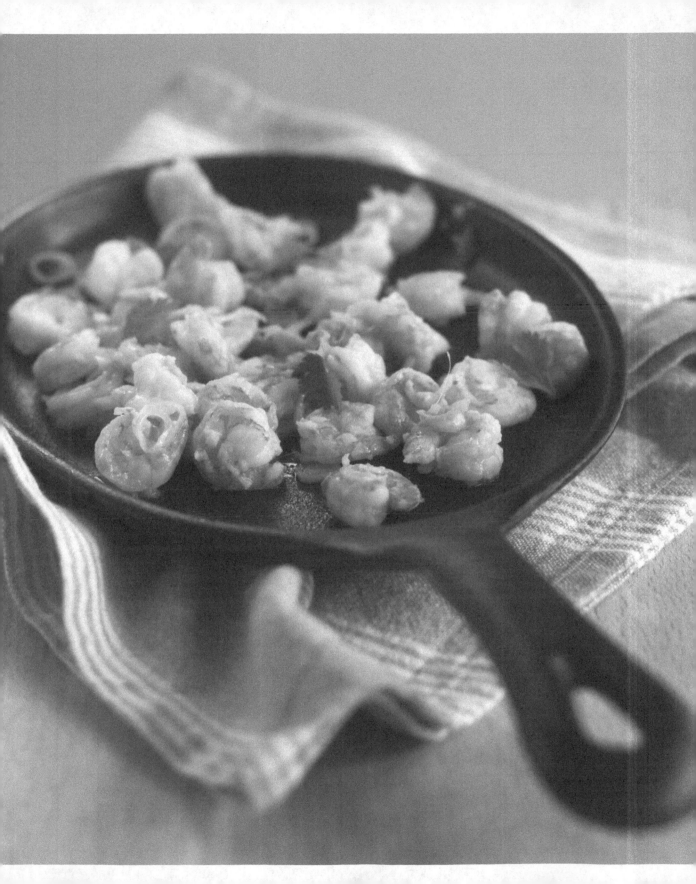

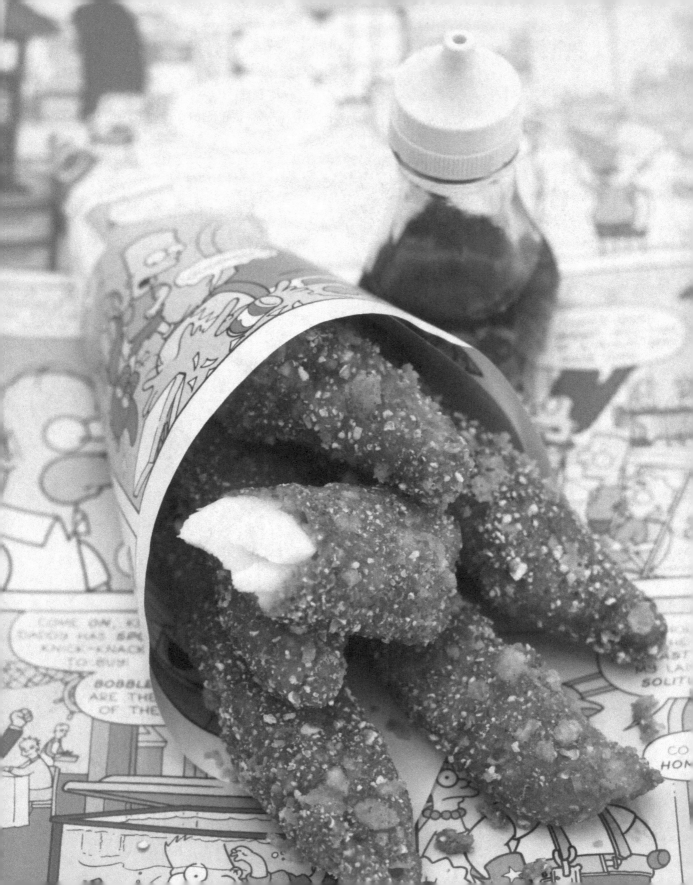

golden fish sticks

Crushed cornflakes make a delicious coating. If you like, you could add a pinch of cayenne pepper. Serve with homemade tartar sauce or just ketchup.

¾ cup cornflakes
½ pound skinless cod fillets (or use flounder or sole)
salt and freshly ground black pepper, to season
2 tablespoons all-purpose flour, for coating
1 egg, lightly beaten
1½ tablespoons canola oil

TARTAR SAUCE
½ cup mayonnaise
fresh lemon juice, to taste
1 tablespoon chopped fresh parsley
1 tablespoon capers, chopped
2 teaspoons chopped gherkins
1 tablespoon snipped fresh chives

* Put the cornflakes in a plastic bag, crush using a rolling pin, and spread out on a plate. Cut the fish into 6 strips and season with salt and pepper. Coat with the flour. Dip in the lightly beaten egg, then coat with the crushed cornflakes.
* Heat the oil in a frying pan and sauté the fish for 3 to 4 minutes until golden and completely cooked, turning halfway through.
* To make the tartar sauce, simply mix together all the sauce ingredients. Serve with the fish sticks.

anything
which
looks at me

crunchy popcorn fish

You don't always have to coat fish in bread crumbs. Why not try to entice kids to eat more fish by coating it with popcorn or potato chips? If using chips, I would use half a large package. If using plain chips, add ½ cup freshly grated Parmesan and some paprika—or use flavored chips. You can use gluten-free flour instead of all-purpose flour. You could serve these with ketchup or tartar sauce (see Golden Fish Sticks, page 81).

2 cups lightly salted popcorn
½ cup grated sharp Cheddar
½ cup freshly grated Parmesan
1 teaspoon paprika
freshly ground black pepper, to season
four 6-ounce skinless cod or salmon fillets
salt, to season
2 tablespoons all-purpose flour, for dusting
2 eggs, beaten with a pinch of salt
2 to 3 tablespoons canola oil, for frying

* Put the popcorn, cheeses, and paprika in a food processor and whiz for 1 to 2 minutes until the popcorn is reduced to crumbs. Season to taste with plenty of pepper, then spread out on a large plate.
* Cut the fish into strips about the size of fish sticks, season with a little salt, dust with the flour, dip in the beaten egg, and coat with the popcorn mixture.
* Heat the oil in a large frying pan and cook the fish over medium heat for 2 to 3 minutes on each side until the coating is crispy and the fish is just cooked. Drain briefly on paper towels before serving.

bag-baked cod niçoise

The flavors of the south of France in individual parcels. Baking
fish in a parcel keeps it wonderfully moist and seals in the flavor.
You might think it strange that I am using olives—my daughter liked
eating olives at the age of two and, surprisingly, they are popular
with quite a few children. If your child doesn't like olives, you could
use four chopped sun-dried tomatoes in olive oil instead.

1 small red onion, diced
1 teaspoon olive oil
1 small garlic clove, crushed
1 teaspoon balsamic vinegar
½ teaspoon sugar
8 ounces cherry tomatoes, quartered
6 or 7 pitted black olives, quartered
salt and freshly ground black pepper, to season
four 6-ounce skinless cod fillets
4 large squares of aluminum foil

12 fresh basil leaves, to serve (optional)

* Sauté the onion in the oil for 7 to 8 minutes until soft. Add the garlic and
balsamic vinegar and cook until the vinegar has evaporated, then stir in the
sugar, tomatoes, and olives and cook for 2 to 3 minutes, until the tomatoes
start to soften. Remove from the heat and season to taste with salt and
pepper. Allow to cool slightly (you can make this in advance and store in
the fridge for up to 2 days).
* Preheat the oven to 400°F. Lay a piece of fish in the center of each foil square
and season with salt and pepper. Put a quarter of the tomato mixture on top
of each piece of fish, then bring the edges of each square of foil together and
scrunch to seal. Put the 4 parcels on a baking sheet and bake for 8 minutes or
until the cod is opaque and starting to flake. Thick pieces of fish may take
2 to 3 minutes longer.
* Serve the fish with the tomato mixture and any juices from the parcel
spooned over the top and garnished with torn basil leaves, if you like.

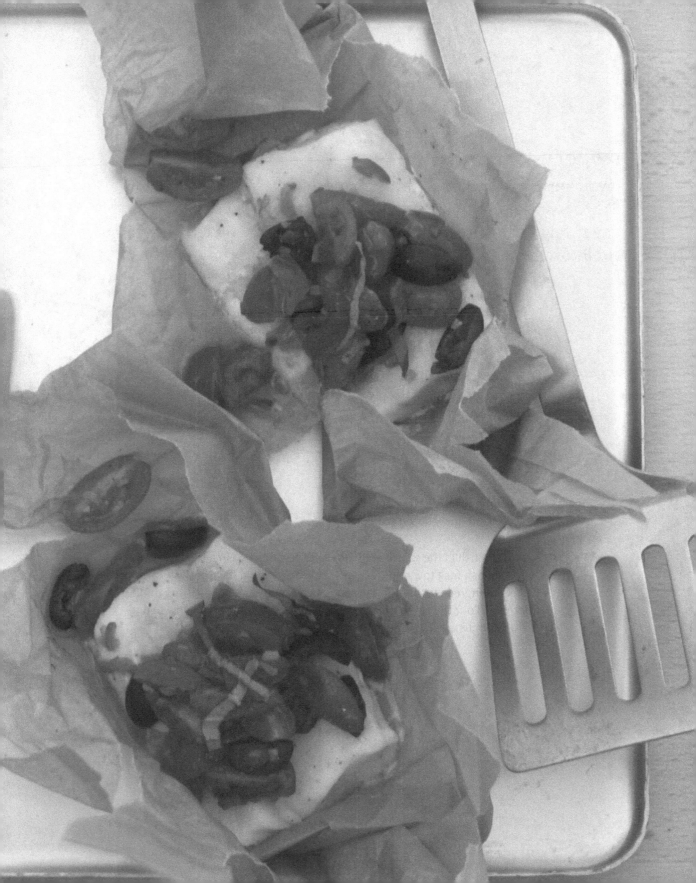

sweet-and-sour fish

If you are having difficulty getting your child to eat fish, you might like to try making this sweet-and-sour sauce. The sauce will mask any strong fishy taste. This would also work using chicken breasts cut into cubes and chicken broth instead of fish broth.

½ pound skinless cod fillet, cut into cubes, or sole fillet, cut into strips
all-purpose flour, seasoned with salt and pepper, for coating
1½ tablespoons canola oil

SWEET-AND-SOUR SAUCE
½ cup fish broth
1 tablespoon white wine vinegar
1 tablespoon superfine sugar
1½ tablespoons ketchup
1½ teaspoons soy sauce
1½ teaspoons cornstarch
1 tablespoon water
½ teaspoon Asian sesame oil
1 tablespoon finely sliced scallion

* Coat the fish in the seasoned flour. Heat the canola oil in a frying pan and sauté the fish for 3 to 4 minutes until cooked (it should flake easily with a fork).
* Mix the ingredients for the sauce and heat gently in a pan, stirring until thickened. Pour the sauce over the fish, heat through, and serve on a bed of fluffy white rice if you like.

drunken fish with little trees

The secret to getting fussy eaters to enjoy eating fish is to come up with a tasty sauce. This Chinese-style sauce is popular with my three children and it takes only a few minutes to prepare. Giving food fun names can encourage children to eat—for instance, "little trees" is a good way to describe broccoli florets. Interestingly, many children who are not keen on other green vegetables do enjoy broccoli.

CHINESE-STYLE SAUCE
1 cup chicken broth
2 teaspoons soy sauce
1 teaspoon Asian sesame oil
1 tablespoon superfine sugar
1 teaspoon cider vinegar
1 tablespoon cornstarch
1 scallion, thinly sliced

5 or 6 broccoli florets
¾ pound skinless flounder fillet, cut into 2-inch strips, or cod fillet
    cut into 1½-inch cubes
3 tablespoons all-purpose flour, seasoned with salt and pepper for cooking
1½ tablespoons canola oil

* To make the sauce, mix together the broth, soy sauce, sesame oil, sugar, vinegar, and cornstarch. Pour the mixture into a saucepan. Bring to a boil, then simmer for 2 to 3 minutes until thickened and smooth. Stir in the scallion.
* Steam the broccoli florets for about 5 minutes until just tender. Meanwhile, toss the fish in the seasoned flour to coat. Heat the canola oil in a frying pan and sauté the fish for a couple of minutes on each side until just cooked.
* Pour the sauce over the fish, add the broccoli florets, and heat through for about a minute before serving.

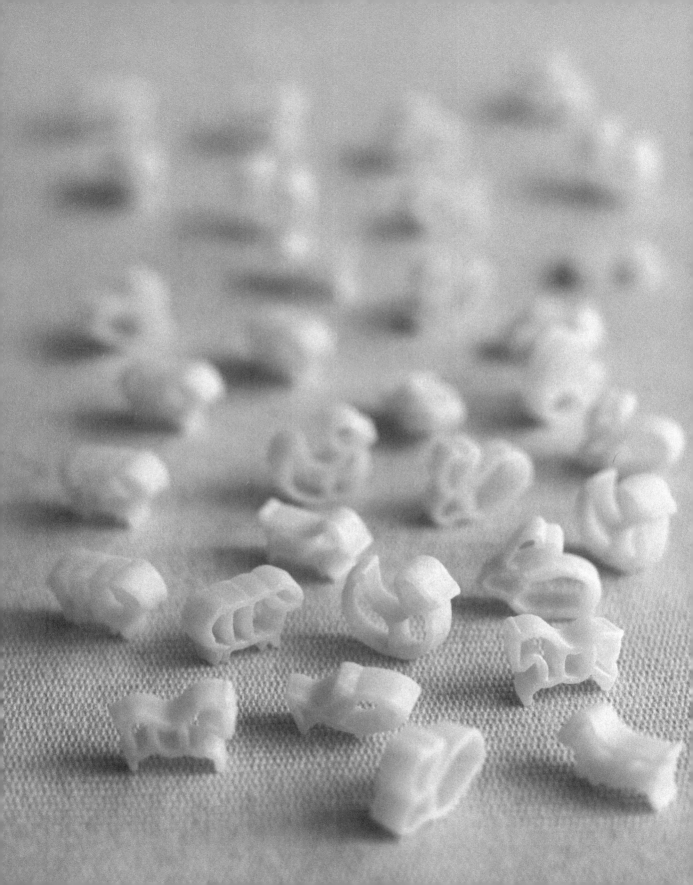

Pasta, please

pork and peanut noodles

If you have a fussy eater who likes peanut butter, try this recipe.
To make life easier, you can buy precooked straight-to-wok rice
noodles, which are really very good, in some supermarkets or in
Asian food stores.

5 ounces thin rice noodles
1 tablespoon canola oil
1 small onion, sliced
1 garlic clove, crushed
½ pound ground pork or chicken
1 cup small snow peas, sliced in half
2 tablespoons crunchy peanut butter
2 teaspoons light brown sugar
1 tablespoon soy sauce
½ cup chicken broth
1 teaspoon seeded finely chopped red chile pepper
a small bunch of fresh cilantro, chopped (optional)

* Place the noodles in a bowl, cover with boiling water, and leave to soak for
5 minutes, then drain. Alternatively, you can use precooked rice noodles.
* Heat the oil in a wok or frying pan, then sauté the onion for 4 minutes. Add
the garlic and cook for 1 minute. Add the pork or chicken and stir-fry for about
8 minutes until the juices have evaporated and the meat is starting to look
crisp. Throw in the snow peas and cook for 2 minutes.
* Meanwhile, mix together the peanut butter, brown sugar, soy sauce, broth,
and chile. Add the peanut sauce and the noodles to the wok or frying pan, toss
well, and stir-fry for about 1 minute until heated through. Before serving, you
could sprinkle with a little cilantro.

PREPARATION TIME 10 MINUTES
COOKING TIME 1 HOUR
MAKES 4 PORTIONS
SAUCE SUITABLE FOR FREEZING

hidden vegetable spaghetti bolognese

This Bolognese sauce sneaks in five vegetables, and it tastes great even to confirmed veggie haters—what you can't see, you can't complain about! You can also use this sauce to make lasagne or shepherd's pie (see pages 96 and 139).

2 tablespoons olive oil
1 small red onion, finely chopped
1 leek, carefully washed and thinly sliced
¾ cup sliced mushrooms
1 medium carrot, grated
½ small celery stalk, diced
1 garlic clove, crushed
⅔ cup beef broth
½ pound ground beef
two 14.5-ounce cans diced tomatoes or canned crushed tomatoes
3 tablespoons tomato paste
1 tablespoon tomato ketchup
1 teaspoon superfine sugar
about 10 ounces spaghetti

* Heat 1 tablespoon of the oil and sauté the onion for 3 minutes. Add the remaining vegetables except the garlic and sauté for 7 minutes. Add the garlic and sauté for 1 minute. Add the broth and simmer for 10 minutes, then blitz the mixture in a food processor.
* Heat the remaining 1 tablespoon oil in a large frying pan and brown the meat for 5 minutes, breaking up well with a fork or wooden spoon. Add the diced tomatoes, tomato paste, ketchup, and sugar and cook for 30 minutes. Add the vegetable puree and continue to cook for 2 minutes more.
* Meanwhile, cook the spaghetti in lightly salted boiling water according to the package directions. Drain and toss with the sauce.

mummy's ramen noodles

Always popular with kids, but the ones you buy are really high in salt. It takes only a few minutes to make your own! It's fun to serve them in a cup.

2½ ounces Chinese-style dried thin egg noodles (lo mein) or use
   bean thread (cellophane) noodles
½ cup chicken broth
1½ teaspoons soy sauce
⅓ cup frozen peas
½ cup drained canned corn or frozen corn
½ cup shredded cooked chicken
½ teaspoon cornstarch
1 scallion, thinly sliced

* Cook the noodles according to the package directions. Drain and set aside. Put the broth, soy sauce, peas, corn, and chicken in a pan over medium heat. Bring to a simmer and cook for 2 minutes.
* In a small cup, mix the cornstarch with 1 teaspoon cold water and add to the contents of the pan, then cook, stirring, for another minute or until the liquid thickens slightly. Add the noodles and scallion and reheat briefly, stirring. Transfer to a bowl or small cup to serve.

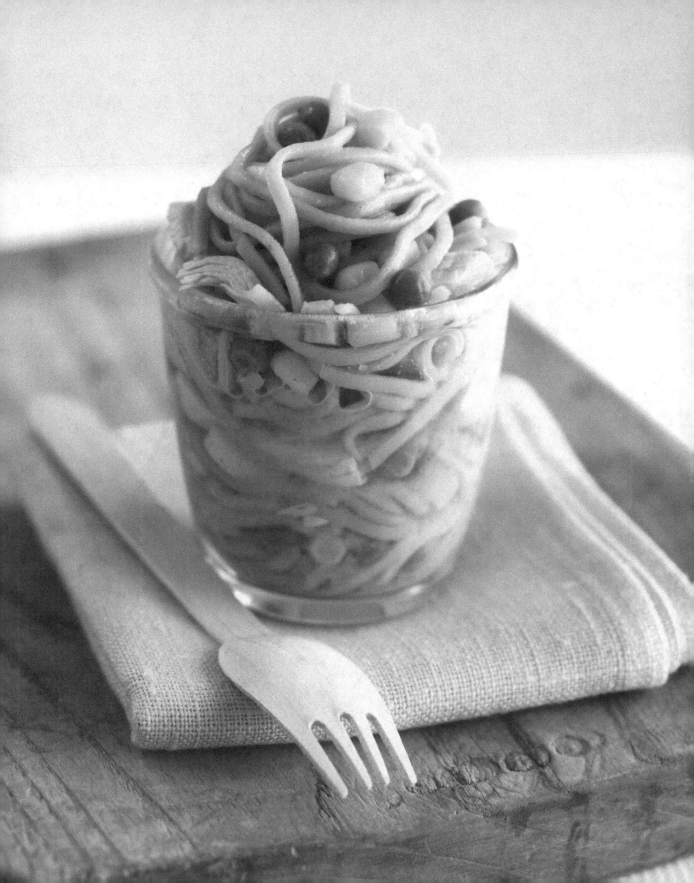

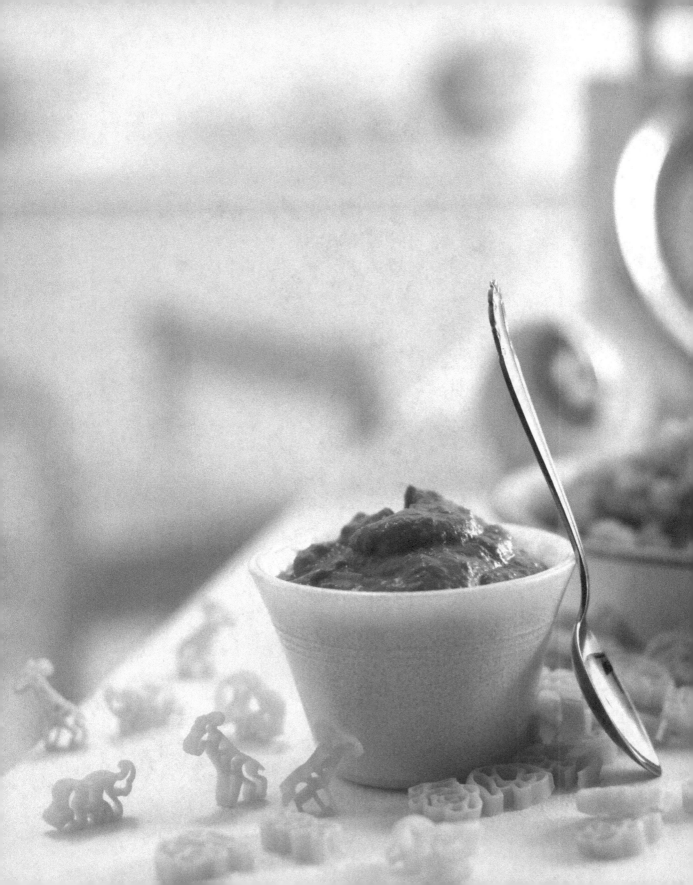

pasta with tomato and mascarpone sauce

My children, like most, prefer pasta with tomato sauce, so I always try to add other ingredients such as chopped vegetables, which I puree into the sauce. It's nice to make a slightly creamy tomato sauce by stirring in some mascarpone cheese. The novelty-shaped pasta adds child interest. This sauce would also be good with steamed white fish or poached chicken.

1 tablespoon olive oil
1 red onion, chopped
¼ cup chopped carrot
¼ cup chopped zucchini
2 tablespoons chopped celery
1 garlic clove, crushed
½ cup sliced button mushrooms
one 15-ounce can tomato sauce (preferably with no added salt)
½ teaspoon sugar
2 tablespoons torn fresh basil leaves (optional)
½ cup mascarpone cheese
salt and freshly ground black pepper, to season
2¼ cups animal-shaped pasta (or any novelty shape)

* Heat the oil in a saucepan and sauté the onion, carrot, zucchini, and celery for 5 minutes. Add the garlic and sauté for 1 minute. Add the mushrooms and sauté for 2 minutes. Stir in the tomato sauce and sugar, and simmer for 10 minutes with the lid on, stirring occasionally.
* Remove from the heat, add the basil, if using, and blend in a food processor. At this point the sauce may be frozen. Return to the pan and add the mascarpone cheese. Simmer for 1 to 2 minutes and stir until the cheese has melted. Season to taste.
* In the meantime, cook the pasta in a large pot of lightly salted boiling water according to the package directions. Drain and toss with the sauce.

PREPARATION TIME 45 MINUTES (1 HOUR IF MAKING
BOLOGNESE SAUCE AS WELL)
COOKING TIME 40 MINUTES (PLUS STANDING TIME)
MAKES 4 PORTIONS
SUITABLE FOR FREEZING

nicholas's lasagne

My son, Nicholas, started out as a fussy eater but now eats absolutely anything. I think he really appreciates home cooking since he has been at university. He comes home most weekends to eat, calling me from the station to ensure that the food will be on the table when he walks in the door! This lasagne is one of his favorites.

BOLOGNESE SAUCE
Hidden Vegetable Bolognese Sauce (page 91)

BÉCHAMEL SAUCE
4 tablespoons (½ stick) butter
½ cup all-purpose flour
2½ cups milk
salt and white pepper, to season
a pinch of grated nutmeg
¼ teaspoon Dijon mustard

9 sheets no-boil lasagne
⅔ cup grated Cheddar
½ cup freshly grated Parmesan

* Prepare the Bolognese sauce.
* Preheat the oven to 400°F. Make the béchamel sauce by melting the butter, then stirring in the flour. Cook for 1 minute, then stir in the milk a little at a time until the sauce is thickened. Bring to a simmer, stirring constantly, and season the sauce well with salt and pepper, a good pinch of nutmeg, and the mustard.
* Spread a quarter of the béchamel in a thin layer in the bottom of a 12 x 7-inch ovenproof dish and add a layer of pasta on top (3 lasagne sheets). Spoon on another quarter of the béchamel and spread it over the pasta, then top with half of the Bolognese. Repeat the pasta, béchamel, Bolognese, then a top layer of pasta, and spoon the remaining béchamel on top. Scatter the cheeses on top and bake for 40 minutes or until piping hot. Allow to stand for 10 minutes before serving.

marina's pasta with pesto and cherry tomatoes

Marina is from the Philippines and has been helping me in the kitchen for more than fifteen years. Not only is she a fabulous cook, but she is also a dear friend and we often spend time testing and inventing recipes together.

½ pound fusilli pasta
2 tablespoons olive oil
1 large onion, sliced
1 garlic clove, crushed
½ pound skinless, boneless chicken breasts, cut into strips
8 ounces cherry tomatoes, halved
3 tablespoons basil or other green pesto
1 tablespoon soy sauce
1 tablespoon balsamic vinegar
salt and freshly ground black pepper, to season
freshly grated Parmesan, to serve (optional)

* Cook the fusilli in lightly salted boiling water according to the package directions. Drain and set aside.
* Heat the oil in a large frying pan or wok. Sauté the onion for 3 minutes, stirring occasionally, then add the garlic and cook for 1 minute. Add the chicken and stir-fry for 2 minutes, then add the cherry tomatoes and stir-fry for another 2 minutes. Add the pesto, soy sauce, and balsamic vinegar and cook for 1 minute. Add the cooked pasta and season to taste with a little salt and pepper and continue to cook for a minute or so until heated through. If you like, you can sprinkle with Parmesan before serving.

☆ I find that quite a few children really like pesto. There is a selection of really good ready-made pestos available in the supermarket, so try adding some to your child's pasta together with fresh ingredients.

fresh tomato sauce for spaghetti

This is one of my children's favorite meals. You will need to choose good-quality, ripe plum tomatoes to get the best flavor—look for ones with a dark red color. Tomatoes are a good source of lycopene, a powerful antioxidant that helps prevent heart disease and cancer. Interestingly, they are better for you cooked in a little oil or butter, as this helps our bodies to absorb the lycopene more efficiently.

2 tablespoons olive oil
2 small onions, chopped
1 fat garlic clove, crushed
10 large plum tomatoes
1 teaspoon sugar
2 tablespoons butter
8 fresh basil leaves, torn into pieces
salt and freshly ground black pepper, to season
½ pound spaghetti
freshly grated Parmesan, to serve (optional)

* Heat the oil and sauté the onions and garlic for 3 minutes. Peel the whole tomatoes by scoring a cross in the bottom of each and placing about 4 at a time in a large pan of boiling water for about 15 seconds. Using a slotted spoon, transfer the tomatoes into a bowl of ice water. When cool enough to handle, remove from the water and pull off the skins using your fingers or a small knife. Seeded tomatoes make thicker sauces—it's easy to remove the seeds using a melon baller or teaspoon.
* Dice the tomatoes and add with the sugar to the onion. Cook for 30 minutes. Stir in the butter and basil leaves and season to taste. Some children are put off if they see green bits in their tomato sauce, so you may want to divide the sauce into two and add basil to only one-half—offer the sauce with the basil first.
* In the meantime, cook the spaghetti in a large pot of lightly salted boiling water according to the package directions. Drain and toss with the sauce. If you like, sprinkle with the Parmesan to serve.

i don't like...

anything
with basil

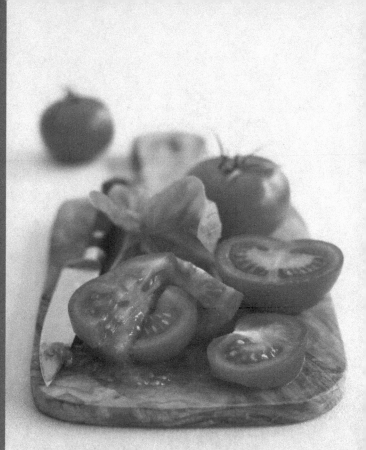

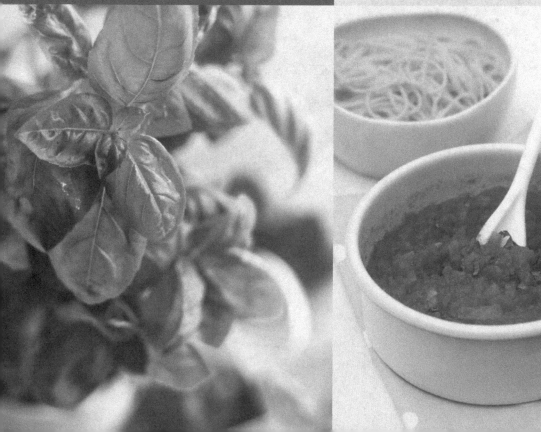

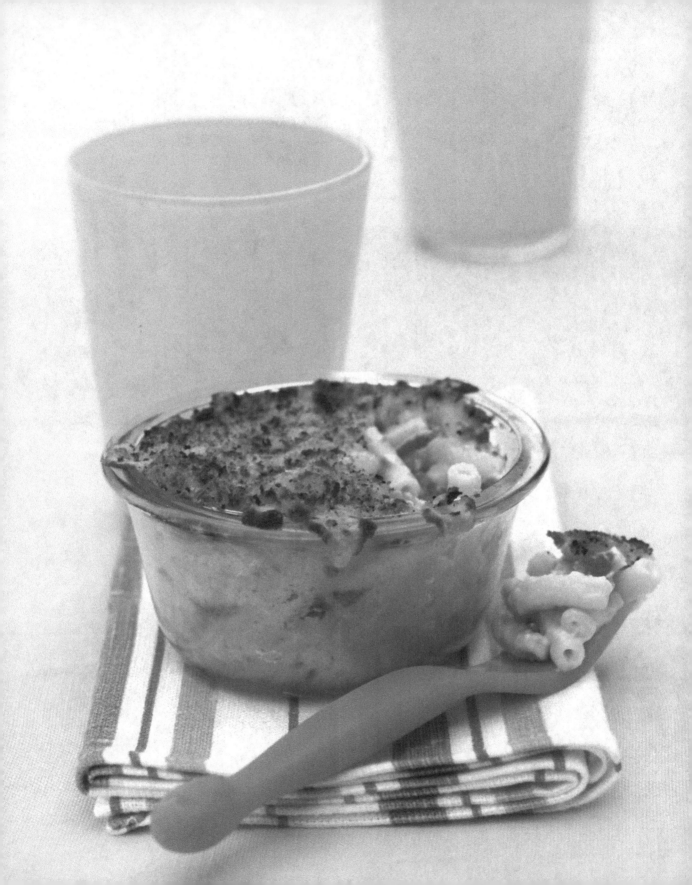

mighty mac and cheese

I know lots of fussy children who only ever want to eat plain pasta with grated cheese. Maybe with a little gentle persuasion they could be enticed to try this tasty macaroni and cheese. You can make it with or without the ham and tomato—it's a really delicious cheese sauce. Pasta is a good source of complex carbohydrates, so this macaroni will boost your child's energy levels as well as providing protein and calcium.

¾ pound macaroni

CHEESE SAUCE
3 tablespoons butter
¼ cup all-purpose flour
2 cups milk
¾ cup grated Gruyère
¼ cup freshly grated Parmesan
¾ cup mascarpone cheese

4 medium tomatoes, peeled, seeded, and chopped (see page 98)
⅓ cup shredded sliced ham (optional)

TOPPING
¾ cup fresh bread crumbs (about 2 slices bread,
   white or whole wheat, crusts removed)
2 tablespoons freshly grated Parmesan

* Cook the pasta in plenty of lightly salted boiling water according to the package directions.
* Melt the butter, stir in the flour, and cook for 1 minute. Gradually add the milk, stirring over low heat for 5 to 6 minutes. Take off the heat, stir in the Gruyère and Parmesan until melted, then the mascarpone cheese.
* Drain the pasta, return to the pan, add the cheese sauce, and heat through gently. Stir in the chopped tomatoes and shredded ham, if using.
* Transfer to a greased ovenproof dish (approximately 9 x 5 inches). Mix together the bread crumbs and Parmesan and sprinkle on top. Place under a preheated broiler until golden and bubbling.

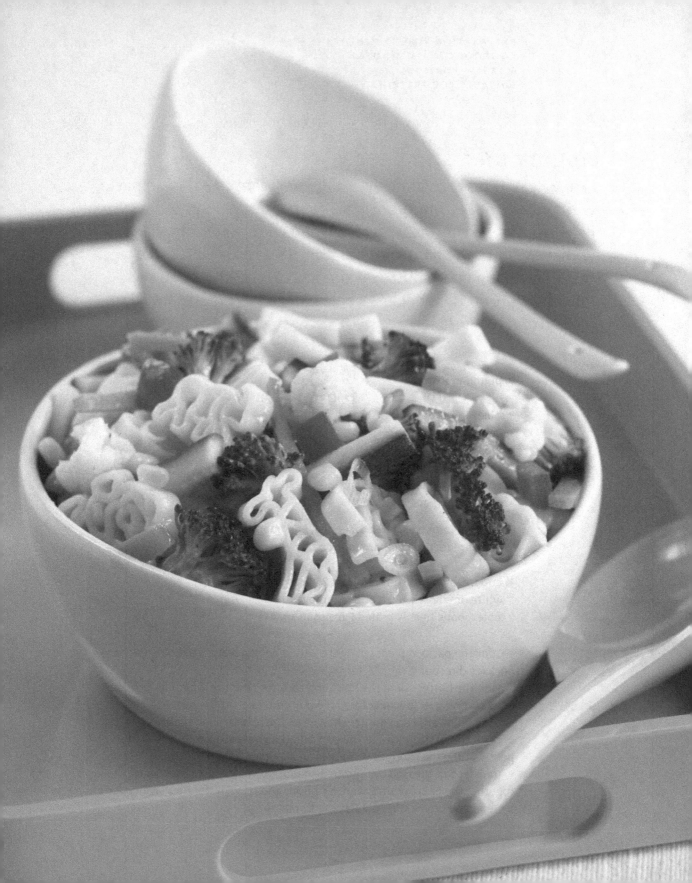

animal pasta salad with multicolored veggies

This can be served warm or cold. It's a good idea to keep a bowl of it in the fridge for your child to snack on during the day. It would also be good as a change from sandwiches in your child's lunch box. You can omit the chicken for vegetarians.

1½ cups animal-shaped pasta (see Note)
1 medium carrot, cut into matchsticks
3 small broccoli florets, cut small
3 small cauliflower florets, cut small
¼ cup string beans, trimmed and cut in half
½ red bell pepper, diced
1 medium to large zucchini, trimmed and cut into matchsticks
⅓ cup drained canned corn
salt and freshly ground black pepper, to season
¼ cup diced cooked chicken (optional)

DRESSING
2 tablespoons cider or red wine vinegar
salt and freshly ground black pepper, to season
⅓ cup olive oil
2 scallions, thinly sliced, or 2 tablespoons snipped fresh chives
½ teaspoon sugar

* Cook the pasta in lightly salted boiling water according to the package directions, drain, and set aside.
* Steam the carrot, broccoli, cauliflower, and beans for 2 minutes. Add the bell pepper and zucchini and continue to cook for another 5 minutes. Add the corn for the last minute. Transfer the vegetables to a serving bowl and season with a little salt and pepper. Stir in the drained pasta and the chicken, if using.
* To make the dressing, whisk the vinegar with the salt and pepper, then whisk in the oil a little at a time. Add the scallions or chives and the sugar. Toss the pasta salad with the dressing.

☆ Novelty pasta shapes tend to be popular with children. You can get them to name the animals as they eat them.

bacon and tomato spaghetti sauce

Fussy children often like bacon. Canadian bacon gives this sauce
a deliciously smoky flavor, but if you prefer you can use regular bacon.
If your children like mushrooms, then add about 1 cup halved button
mushrooms and broil with the bacon.

8 slices Canadian bacon, cut into 1-inch pieces
two 14.5-ounce cans diced tomatoes
½ teaspoon dried oregano
½ teaspoon sugar
a pinch of red pepper flakes (optional)
10 ounces spaghetti
salt and freshly ground black pepper, to season
freshly grated Parmesan, to serve

* Preheat the broiler. Line a baking sheet with foil. Broil the bacon for 2 to 3
minutes on each side, until crisp. Mix together the tomatoes, oregano, sugar,
and red pepper flakes, if using, and pour on top of the bacon. Broil for another
8 to 10 minutes, stirring 3 or 4 times, until the sauce has thickened slightly and
is bubbling.
* Meanwhile, cook the spaghetti in lightly salted boiling water according to the
package directions and drain well. Season the sauce with pepper but go easy on
the salt, as bacon is usually quite salty. Serve the spaghetti with the sauce
spooned over it and sprinkled with grated Parmesan.

kiddie carbonara

A quick and easy way to make a super pasta sauce. Tailor it to your child's taste by adding different vegetables or even diced cooked chicken or shrimp instead of the ham.

6 ounces pasta (fusilli, bow ties, or spaghetti)
½ cup frozen peas
1 tablespoon crème fraîche or sour cream
2 tablespoons fresh lemon juice
2 tablespoons freshly grated Parmesan, plus a little to serve
2 to 4 slices ham, cut into strips
salt and freshly ground black pepper, to season

* Cook the pasta in lightly salted boiling water according to the package directions, adding the peas for the last 2 minutes of cooking time. Reserve a cupful of cooking water, then drain the pasta and return it to the pan.
* Stir the crème fraîche, lemon juice, and Parmesan into the pasta. Add a splash of the cooking water if it becomes too dry. Stir in the ham. Season to taste and serve with the extra Parmesan.

caroline's lasagne alfredo

Lasagne tends to be popular with children, so it's a good idea to combine the pasta itself with some other nutritious ingredients. This delicious lasagne is made with chicken and spinach. You can use the dried no-boil variety or fresh lasagne—I prefer fresh.

ALFREDO SAUCE
5 tablespoons butter
1 small onion, finely chopped
1 garlic clove, crushed
½ cup all-purpose flour
1½ cups chicken broth
1¼ cups milk
1 cup grated Cheddar
½ cup freshly grated Parmesan (reserve ¼ cup for the topping)
salt and freshly ground black pepper, to season
freshly grated nutmeg, to season

8 ounces fresh spinach, carefully washed
9 sheets no-boil lasagne
2 boneless, skinless chicken breasts, about 4 ounces each, thinly sliced
salt and freshly ground black pepper, to season

* Melt the butter in a medium pan and sauté the onion for 5 to 6 minutes until soft and just starting to turn golden. Add the garlic and cook for 1 minute, then stir in the flour and cook for 1 minute. Remove from the heat and gradually stir in the broth and milk. Cook over medium heat, stirring constantly, until the sauce thickens and comes to a simmer. Remove from the heat, allow to cool for a minute, then stir in the Cheddar and ½ cup of the Parmesan and season well with salt, pepper, and nutmeg.
* Cook the spinach in a large dry pan until wilted. Allow to cool, then squeeze out as much liquid as possible and chop roughly.
* Preheat the oven to 400°F. Put a thin layer of sauce in the bottom of a 9 x 5-inch ovenproof dish and add a layer of 3 lasagne sheets. Scatter half of the spinach and chicken on top, season with salt and pepper, and spoon one-third of the sauce on top. Add another layer of 3 lasagne, and repeat layers of spinach, chicken, seasoning, sauce, and 3 lasagne. Top with the remaining sauce and sprinkle the reserved Parmesan on top. Bake for 40 to 45 minutes or until piping hot in the center. Allow to stand for 15 minutes before serving.

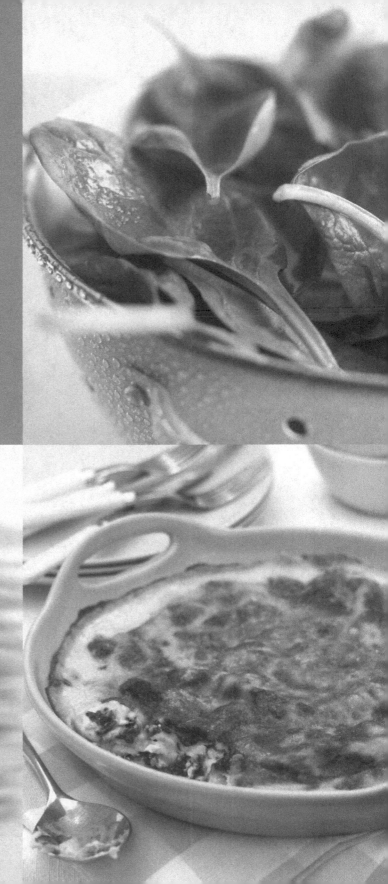

i don't like...

anything

green

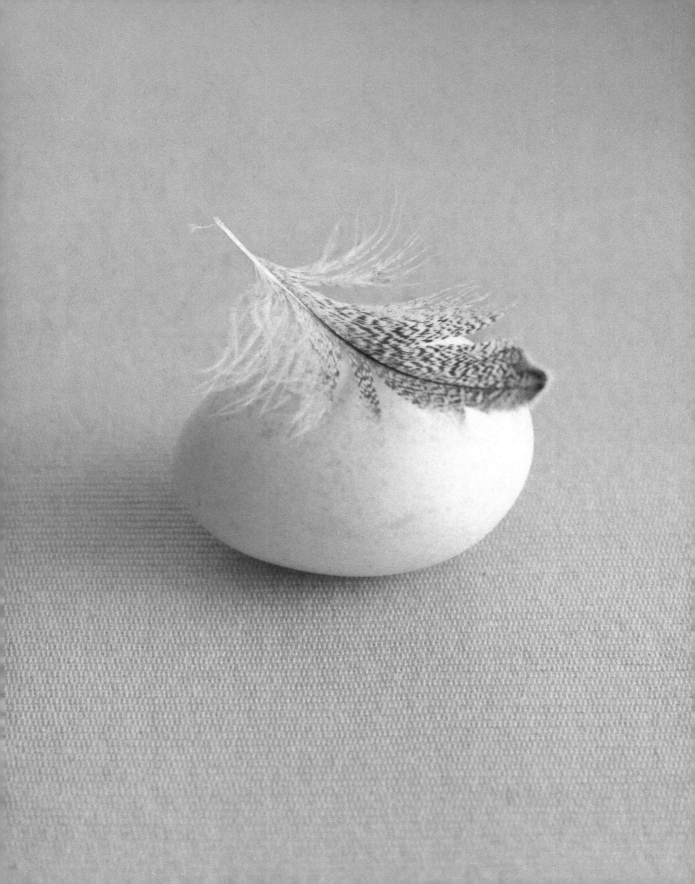

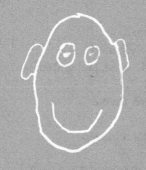

cheeky chicken

mini chicken patties

My Chicken and Apple Balls recipe in my first book, *The Healthy Baby Meal Planner*, was created for my son, Nicholas. He liked apples but wouldn't eat chicken, so I combined the two and made Chicken and Apple Ball finger food. It's good to find finger foods for children that are also nutritious, and the apple combines with the chicken, giving it a lovely flavor and keeping it really moist.

½ red onion, finely chopped
½ medium carrot, coarsely grated
½ medium apple, peeled, cored, and grated
3 tablespoons canola oil
½ teaspoon chopped fresh thyme
1 garlic clove, crushed
1 slice white bread, crusts removed
½ pound ground chicken
½ crumbled chicken bouillon cube (optional)
salt and freshly ground black pepper, to season

* In a large frying pan, sauté the onion, carrot, and apple in 1 tablespoon of the oil for 4 minutes. Stir in the thyme and garlic and cook for 1 minute. Remove from the heat and allow to cool slightly.
* Meanwhile, put the bread in a food processor and whiz into crumbs. Add the onion mixture, chicken, and crumbled bouillon cube (if using) and combine for 1 to 2 minutes. Season to taste. (If you wish, form into patties and freeze.)
* Wipe out the frying pan with paper towels, then add the remaining 2 tablespoons oil. Over medium heat, drop tablespoonfuls of the chicken mixture into the pan, flattening the patties slightly with a spatula or the back of a fork until about ¼ inch thick. Fry for about 1½ minutes on each side in batches of 6 to 8 until golden brown and cooked through. These are good cooked on a grill pan. Drain briefly on paper towels before serving.

☆ To freeze, put the patties on a baking sheet lined with plastic wrap. Cover with more wrap and freeze until solid. When frozen, transfer to a freezer bag.

japanese-style chicken fillets

My kids like to eat this with edamame beans, which are being hailed as the new superfood and look like a cross between a fava bean and a pea. You can buy edamame beans frozen. Lightly boil the pods in salted water and squeeze the seeds into your mouth. I make a dip for the edamame that consists of 2 tablespoons of soy sauce mixed with half a tablespoon of mirin.

3 tablespoons all-purpose flour
2 eggs, lightly beaten
⅓ cup fresh white bread crumbs
1 pound boneless, skinless chicken breasts
salt and freshly ground black pepper, to season

SAUCE
1 medium onion, thinly sliced
1 tablespoon canola oil
4 scallions, thinly sliced
2 tablespoons soy sauce
⅓ cup mirin
1½ cups chicken broth

2 tablespoons canola oil, for frying

* Put the flour, eggs, and bread crumbs into three shallow bowls. Cover the chicken breasts with plastic wrap, then pound with a mallet until about ½ inch thick. Cut each one into 4 strips. Season with salt and pepper, then dip into the flour, then the egg, and finally the bread crumbs.
* To make the sauce, gently fry the onion in the canola oil, covered, for about 5 minutes until very soft, then uncovered for 5 minutes more. Add the scallions, soy sauce, mirin, and broth. Simmer for 3 minutes.
* Fry the chicken strips in batches in the canola oil until golden and cooked through. Serve on a bed of rice with the sauce poured over.

☆ Ethnic-type recipes often work well with fussy children. I use mirin, a sweet Japanese cooking wine, quite a bit. It has a flavor that children like and is the key ingredient in teriyaki sauce (see also Teriyaki Beef Skewers on page 142).

chinese chicken wraps

A tasty tortilla filling with an Asian flavor—I like the scrumptious mix of the mayonnaise and plum sauce and the crunch of the bean sprouts. It might be fun to get your child involved in helping to assemble these. Even small children can help to mix up the filling.

2 tablespoons mayonnaise
1 tablespoon plum sauce
½ teaspoon soy sauce
½ teaspoon fresh lemon juice
a small handful of bean sprouts
½ cup drained canned corn
½ cup shredded cooked chicken
one 7-inch flour tortilla

* Mix together the mayonnaise, plum sauce, soy sauce, and lemon juice. Stir in the bean sprouts, corn, and chicken.
* Heat the tortilla for a few seconds in a microwave or a dry frying pan.
* Arrange the filling near one edge of the tortilla, then roll up. Cut the tortilla in half diagonally. You will need to wrap the end of each half in foil, as the filling is quite wet and will otherwise slip out.

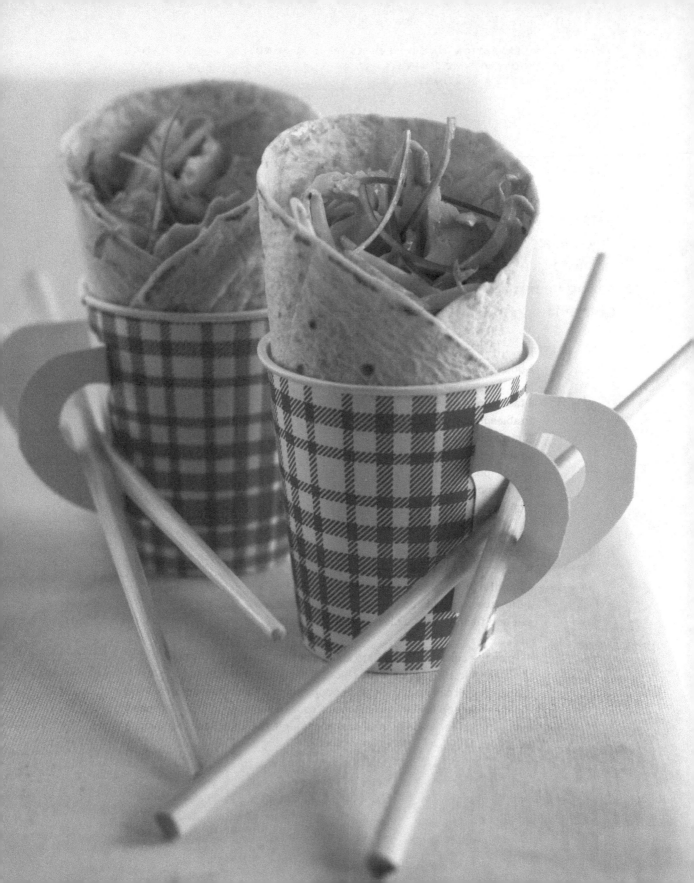

lara's chicken wraps

This is my daughter Lara's favorite recipe. Just like many children, she gets fixated on one particular recipe and would like to eat it every day. She also enjoys assembling the wrap herself. I think that being involved in making their own food can encourage fussy eaters to try eating new things. You could also use strips of Maple-Glazed Grilled Chicken (page 120) inside these wraps.

2 boneless, skinless chicken breasts

MARINADE
1 tablespoon olive oil
1 tablespoon fresh lemon juice
1 garlic clove, lightly crushed
1 tablespoon soy sauce
1 tablespoon honey
1½ teaspoons brown sugar
2 tablespoons canola oil

1 tablespoon canola oil
four 7-inch flour tortillas
¼ cup mayonnaise
a handful of shredded iceberg lettuce
4 tomatoes, seeded and cut into strips
salt and freshly ground black pepper, to season

* Score the chicken with a sharp knife. Mix together all the ingredients for the marinade and marinate the chicken for about 30 minutes.
* Brush a grill pan with the 1 tablespoon canola oil. Remove the chicken from the marinade, and when the pan is hot, cook the chicken for approximately 4 minutes on each side or until cooked through. Then cut into strips and set aside.

* Heat each tortilla for 10 seconds in a microwave or in a hot dry frying pan for 15 seconds, one at a time. Spread each one with 1 tablespoon of the mayonnaise and arrange chicken strips in a line down one side of the tortilla, about 1½ inches from the edge. Place parallel lines of shredded lettuce down one side and tomato strips down the other. Season to taste. Roll up and cut each tortilla in half and wrap in foil to serve.

☆ You can marinate and cook the chicken in advance if you like. If you don't have time to cook the chicken, you can buy some marinated cooked chicken and use that instead.

PREPARATION TIME 5 MINUTES
COOKING TIME 10 MINUTES
MAKES 4 PORTIONS

ten-minute chicken noodle soup

Children tend to like chicken noodle soup, so here's a quick and easy version for you to make at home.

1 medium carrot, diced
4 cups good-quality chicken broth
½ teaspoon chopped fresh thyme leaves
2 ounces thin noodles (such as vermicelli), broken into pieces
⅔ cup shredded cooked chicken
¼ cup frozen peas
salt and freshly ground black pepper, to season

* Put the carrot, broth, and thyme in a medium pan. Bring to a boil and add the noodles. Simmer for 5 minutes or until the noodles are just cooked.
* Add the chicken and frozen peas. Bring back to a simmer and cook for another minute. Season to taste.

i don't like...

naked chicken
without bread crumbs

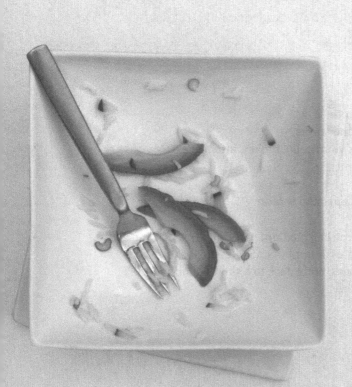

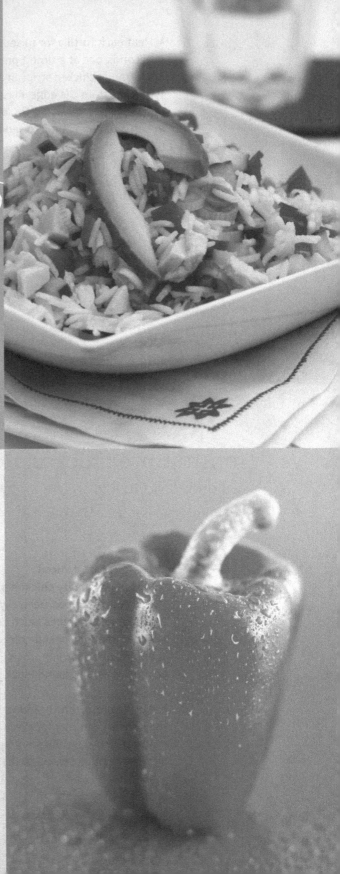

japanese chicken salad

A delicious chicken salad made with Thai jasmine rice. You can buy this in most supermarkets—it's quite similar to sushi rice. The crunchy texture of the cucumber and red bell pepper contrasts well with the rice, and the dressing gives the salad a delicious flavor that is not too strong, so it should attract fussy eaters. This would make a good addition to your child's lunch box.

½ cup Thai jasmine rice

DRESSING
2 tablespoons rice wine vinegar
1 tablespoon superfine sugar
1½ teaspoons canola oil

⅓ large cucumber, preferably English or hothouse
3 scallions, sliced
½ red bell pepper, diced
¾ cup diced cooked chicken
¼ avocado, sliced (optional)
salt and freshly ground black pepper, to season

* Put the rice in a large pan with 1½ cups cold water and a pinch of salt. Bring to a boil and simmer for 12 to 15 minutes until the rice is just tender. Drain and leave to stand in a sieve for 15 minutes, stirring halfway through, then transfer to a bowl.
* To make the dressing, gently warm the rice wine vinegar and sugar until the sugar has dissolved. Add the canola oil and stir into the rice. Leave until room temperature and refrigerate (if using for a lunch box).
* Cut the cucumber in half lengthwise and scoop out the seeds with a teaspoon. Dice the flesh. Stir into the dressed rice with the scallions, bell pepper, chicken, and avocado, if using, and season to taste.

nasi goreng: indonesian fried rice

Indonesians use kecap manis, a sweetened soy sauce. If you have this, then use 3 tablespoons rather than the soy sauce and brown sugar. You can add extra vegetables with the bell pepper, such as broccoli florets or snow peas.

2 eggs
salt and freshly ground black pepper, to season
1 tablespoon canola oil
1 medium onion, thinly sliced
¼ red bell pepper, diced
1 garlic clove, crushed
½ teaspoon grated fresh ginger
3 cups cold cooked rice (1 cup uncooked)
½ cup frozen peas
1½ to 1¾ cups shredded cooked chicken
¼ cup cooked peeled small shrimp
2 tablespoons soy sauce
1 tablespoon light brown sugar
4 small or 2 large scallions, thinly sliced
a handful of fresh cilantro leaves, to serve (optional)
1 lime, quartered, to serve (optional)

* Beat the eggs with a pinch of salt and a few grindings of black pepper. Heat 1 teaspoon of the oil in a wok and when sizzling, add the eggs to make an omelet. Cook for 1 to 2 minutes (the eggs may puff a bit), until golden on the underside, then flip the omelet over and cook for another minute or until set. Transfer to a plate and cut into small pieces.
* Heat the remaining 2 teaspoons oil in the wok and stir-fry the onion for 4 minutes. Add the bell pepper, garlic, and ginger, and cook for another 2 to 3 minutes until the onion is golden. Add the cooked rice, peas, chicken, and shrimp and stir-fry for another 5 minutes, until everything is hot.
* Mix the soy sauce and brown sugar together and stir through the rice, along with the pieces of omelet. Remove from the heat and stir in the scallions. Serve with the cilantro leaves scattered on top and the lime wedges to squeeze over.

monday-night risotto

In my house this is often known as Monday-Night Risotto, as it is a good way to use up leftover roast chicken. This method gives a deliciously creamy risotto.

4 tablespoons (½ stick) butter
2 large shallots or 2 small onions, finely chopped
1 garlic clove, crushed
1 cup risotto rice (such as arborio)
5¼ cups chicken broth, plus more as necessary
1 cup shredded cooked chicken
1 cup frozen peas
¼ cup freshly grated Parmesan, plus extra to serve
¼ teaspoon grated lemon zest
2 tablespoons fresh lemon juice
1½ teaspoons chopped flat-leaf parsley (optional)
salt and freshly ground black pepper, to season

* Melt the butter in a 3-quart saucepan and gently cook the shallots or onions for 5 minutes or until soft but not colored. Add the garlic and rice and cook for 2 minutes or until the rice starts to turn translucent.
* Meanwhile, put the broth in a large saucepan and bring to a boil. Keep on very low heat while you are making the risotto. Add the hot broth to the rice a ladleful at a time, allowing the rice to absorb all the broth before adding any more. Continue to add the broth gradually, stirring often, for about 20 minutes (it might take a little longer) until the rice is tender and creamy but the grains are still firm in the center. Make sure you have some broth left in the pan (about ¼ cup).
* Add the chicken, peas, and Parmesan and cook, stirring, for 2 minutes. Mix in the lemon zest and juice plus enough of the remaining broth to give a loose but not sloppy consistency. Add extra broth if necessary, as the absorption will differ according to the type of rice.
* Remove from the heat and stir in the parsley, then season to taste with salt and pepper. Serve with the extra grated Parmesan.

maple-glazed grilled chicken

This slightly sweet combination of ketchup, maple syrup, and smoked paprika should tempt fussy eaters. The paprika gives the chicken a rich flavor and orange hue. Smoked sweet paprika is available in some supermarkets, through online retailers, and in specialty stores. Be careful not to use hot paprika by mistake!

4 boneless, skinless chicken breasts
MARINADE
5 tablespoons canola oil
¼ cup ketchup
3 tablespoons maple syrup
1 tablespoon smoked sweet paprika

olive oil, for grilling

* First, flatten the chicken. One good way to do so is to slit one side of a plastic freezer bag so that you can position the meat inside, then cover with the plastic. Use a heavy smooth-sided mallet to pound the chicken, working from the middle outward, to a uniform thickness. Or cover with plastic wrap and bash a few times with a mallet.
* Whisk together the canola oil, ketchup, maple syrup, and paprika, pour over the chicken, and leave to marinate for a couple of hours in the fridge.
* Heat a grill pan, brush with a little olive oil, and grill the chicken for about 4 minutes on each side until cooked through, basting occasionally. Pour any pan juices on top to serve.

☆ I like to cook marinated chicken on the grill. A grill is a healthy way of cooking, as it uses little fat and keeps the chicken tender and moist. You can also grill vegetables, such as sliced zucchini, snow peas, and bell peppers. You could use an ordinary grill pan, but one of the best pieces of kitchen equipment that I have is a contact grill. I use it all the time—it functions as an open griddle, an open indoor grill, a contact grill, and a panini press, and it works for everything from chicken and hamburgers to fish and vegetables. It grills both sides of the chicken at once, cutting the cooking time in half.

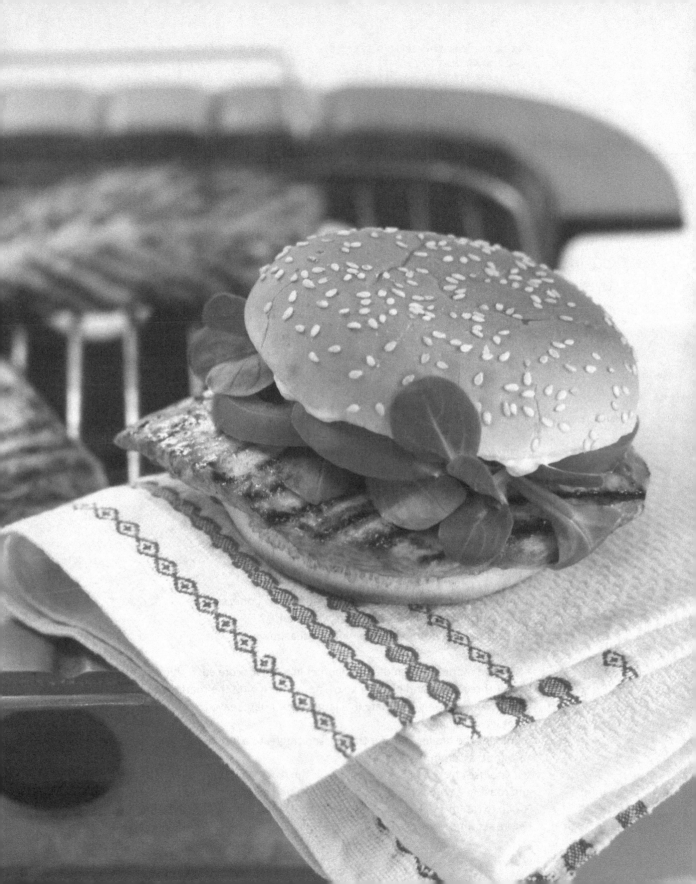

sticky chicken

Mrs. Ball started making chutney from her mother's secret recipe when she moved from Canada to Johannesburg with her seven children. Her friends and family loved it so much that her chutney business went from selling about twenty-four bottles a day in 1918 to over eight thousand bottles a day within only a few years. Mrs. Ball died in 1962 at the age of ninety-seven. Her grandson believes she would have lived to be a hundred if she hadn't been assaulted and robbed by three youths five years earlier as she sat on her front porch in Fish Hoek, near Cape Town.

MARINADE

½ cup Mrs Ball's Original Recipe Chutney (available through on-line specialty
   retailers) or other good-quality mild peach and apricot chutney
2 tablespoons fresh lemon juice
2 tablespoons Worcestershire sauce
2 tablespoons soy sauce
¼ cup ketchup
1 tablespoon honey
2 tablespoons olive oil

8 chicken thighs (about 2½ pounds total), on the bone, skin on,
   or 4 chicken breasts, on the bone, with skin
salt and freshly ground black pepper, to season

* Mix the marinade ingredients together in a bowl. Score each chicken thigh two or three times and place in an ovenproof dish. Add the marinade and season. Alternatively, marinate in a large freezer bag. Leave to marinate for at least 30 minutes.
* Preheat the broiler. Transfer the chicken thighs to a broiler rack and cook for 30 minutes, turning every 5 minutes.
* If you use chicken breasts, marinate in the usual way, then cover with foil and roast at 400°F for 20 minutes. Uncover and cook for another 20 minutes. For an extra-crispy skin, pop under the broiler for a final couple of minutes before serving.

chicken satay skewers

This is a good recipe if you have fussy eaters who like peanut butter—they will appreciate the flavor, and it's fun eating chicken off a skewer. It is also good made with chicken thigh meat, as it's moist and tender, so you could substitute two large chicken thighs for the chicken breast.

MARINADE
1 tablespoon peanut butter
1 tablespoon cream of coconut
½ teaspoon medium curry paste (such as Patak's Balti if available)
1 teaspoon fresh lime juice
a large pinch of salt or ¼ teaspoon fish sauce
¼ teaspoon sugar
1 tablespoon water

6 bamboo skewers, soaked in water for 20 minutes
1 large boneless, skinless chicken breast, cut into ½-inch cubes

* Put the marinade ingredients in a bowl and mix to combine. Add the chicken and toss to coat. Marinate for at least 1 hour and preferably overnight in the fridge.
* Preheat the broiler. Thread 4 or 5 pieces of chicken onto each skewer. Broil for 3 to 4 minutes on each side until cooked through. Alternatively, cook on a grill pan or an outdoor grill.

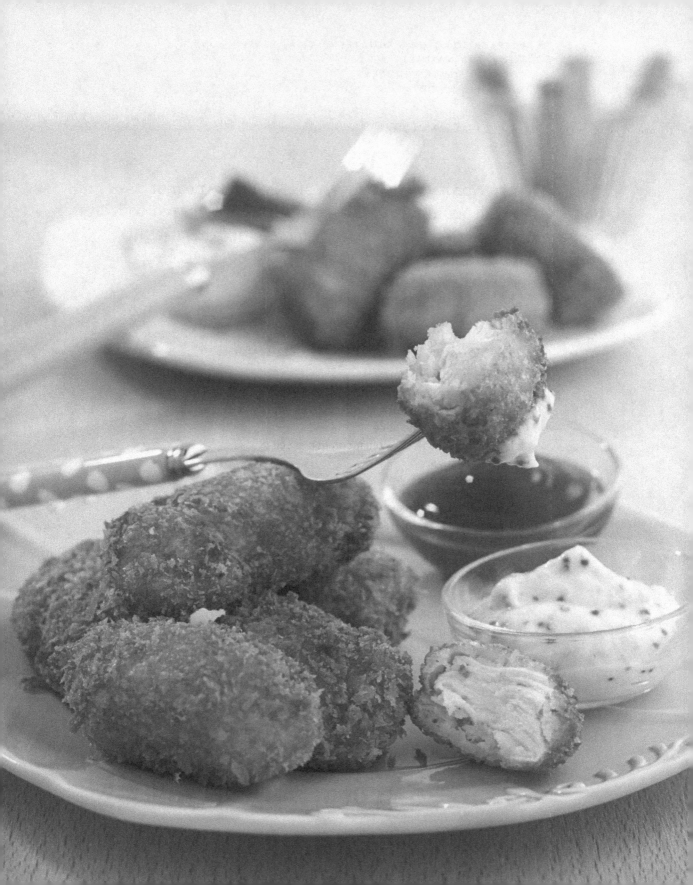

chicken nuggets with dipping sauces

Japanese honey panko bread crumbs are particularly good for this. You can buy these in Asian food stores or some large supermarkets. Otherwise, use plain dried bread crumbs. Marinating chicken in buttermilk gives it a delicious flavor and keeps it nice and tender. Get the kids to help whip up the dips.

MARINADE

1 cup buttermilk
1 tablespoon fresh lemon juice
1 teaspoon Worcestershire sauce
1 teaspoon soy sauce
¼ teaspoon paprika

¾ pound boneless, skinless chicken breasts (about 3 chicken breasts), cut into 1-inch cubes
¼ cup canola oil, for frying

COATING

¾ cup all-purpose flour
1 egg
salt and freshly ground black pepper, to season

¾ cup dried bread crumbs or 1 cup honey panko bread crumbs
⅓ cup freshly grated Parmesan

* Combine the marinade ingredients and soak the chicken cubes for 2 hours.
* Put the flour on a large plate. Beat the egg with 1 tablespoon water and season with salt and pepper. Mix the bread crumbs and Parmesan on a large plate. Remove the chicken cubes from the marinade, shaking off any excess, and toss them in the flour. Then dip the cubes in the egg mixture and roll in the bread crumbs.

* Heat the oil in a large frying pan and sauté the chicken nuggets for 2 to 3 minutes on each side until golden and cooked through, turning occasionally. Alternatively, preheat the oven to 400°F. Put the chicken nuggets on a generously oiled large baking sheet and bake for 18 to 20 minutes until the coating is crisp and the chicken cooked.
* While the nuggets are cooking, you can whip up these easy dips by simply mixing the ingredients in a bowl:

BBQ DIP

⅓ cup ketchup
2 tablespoons maple syrup
½ teaspoon Worcestershire sauce
½ teaspoon soy sauce
2 or 3 drops Tabasco sauce (optional)

HONEY-MUSTARD DIP

¼ cup mayonnaise
1 teaspoon whole-grain Dijon mustard
1½ teaspoons honey
1 teaspoon cold water

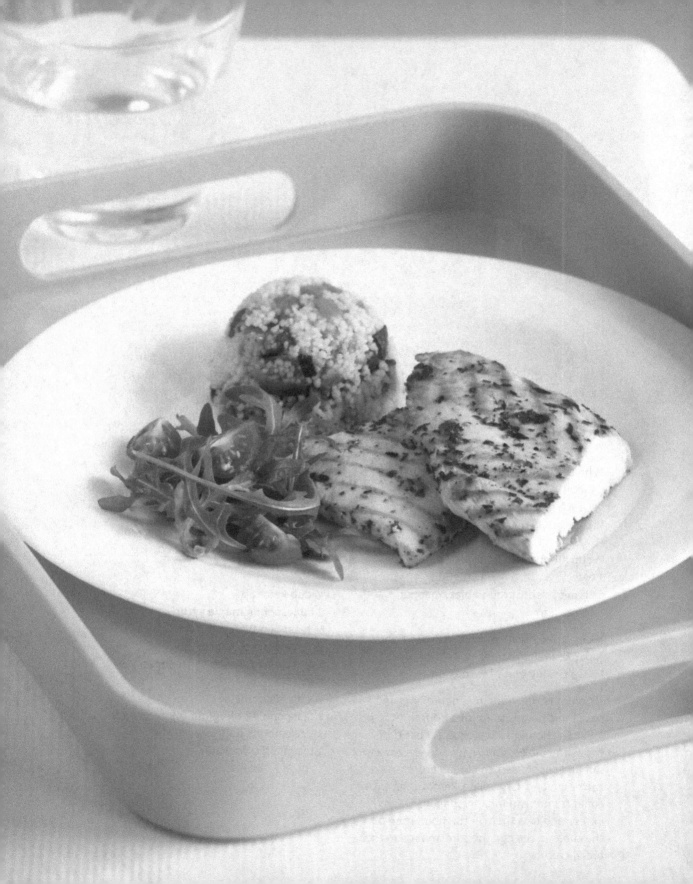

PREPARATION TIME 10 MINUTES (PLUS AT LEAST 20 MINUTES
    FOR MARINATING)
COOKING TIME 8 MINUTES
MAKES 2 PORTIONS

chicken paillard with arugula and cherry tomatoes

I do quite a lot of work with restaurants, trying to introduce healthier meals for children. This is one of the dishes available at London's Villandry, a food store with restaurants, where I have helped design the children's menu. It's very popular, which just goes to show that chicken doesn't always have to be covered in bread crumbs.

2 boneless, skinless chicken breasts

MARINADE
1 garlic clove, finely chopped
1 teaspoon finely chopped fresh thyme
2 tablespoons olive oil
salt and freshly ground black pepper, to season

a little olive oil, for grilling

DRESSING
1 tablespoon olive oil
1 teaspoon balsamic vinegar
a pinch of sugar
salt and freshly ground black pepper, to season

a small bunch of arugula
8 cherry tomatoes, quartered

* Put the chicken breasts between two sheets of plastic wrap or waxed paper and flatten to a ¼-inch thickness with a mallet. Whisk together the garlic, thyme, olive oil, and seasoning, and marinate the chicken in it for at least 20 minutes.
* Heat a grill pan and brush with a little oil. Remove the chicken from the marinade and cook for about 4 minutes on each side until cooked through. If you have a contact grill, you can close the lid and cook the chicken on both sides at the same time, cutting the cooking time in half.
* To make the dressing, combine the olive oil and balsamic vinegar and season with a little sugar, salt, and pepper. Toss with the arugula and cherry tomatoes and serve as a side dish to the chicken.

yummy chicken quesadillas

A quesadilla is what you get when you cook ingredients inside a tortilla. The filling can be wrapped inside by folding the tortilla over, or it can be sandwiched between two tortillas, as in the Vegetable Quesadillas on page 50. I find that children tend to eat food that they would otherwise never eat if it's inside tortillas.

1½ teaspoons canola oil
1 boneless, skinless chicken breast, sliced into small strips
½ onion, sliced
¼ red bell pepper, cut into thin slices
1 tablespoon balsamic vinegar
½ teaspoon brown sugar
2 tablespoons salsa
two 7-inch flour tortillas
½ cup grated Cheddar

* Preheat the broiler. Heat the oil in a wok or large frying pan and stir-fry the chicken for 2 minutes. Add the onion and cook for 2 minutes. Add the bell pepper and cook for 2 to 3 minutes. Add the balsamic vinegar and sugar and cook for 1 minute.

* Spread 1 tablespoon of the salsa over half of each tortilla and sprinkle 2 tablespoons of the Cheddar on top. Divide the chicken mixture between the two tortillas and sprinkle with the remaining ¼ cup cheese. Roll up and secure with a toothpick.

* Broil for 1½ to 2 minutes on each side to warm the tortillas and melt the cheese.

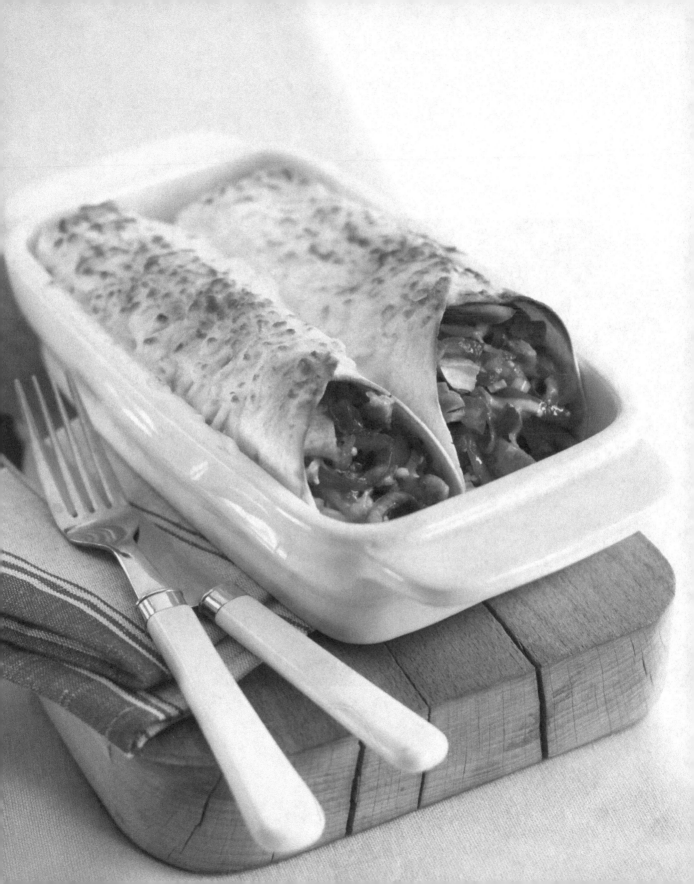

yummy chicken quesadillas ☺

TIP

A hungry child is a less fussy child, so time snacks so that they are not too close to mealtimes. When they come home from school, children are usually starving, so have some good food prepared like these enchiladas (page 128) instead of giving them chips or chocolate cookies.

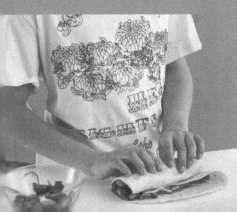

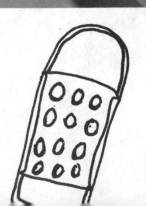

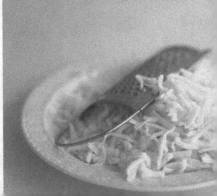

chicken in tomato and sweet pepper sauce

This is a delicious sauce that goes really well with chicken. The red onions and roasted red bell peppers add a sweetness that children like. Serve with fluffy white rice.

2 large red bell peppers, seeded and cored
2 medium red onions, chopped
1 garlic clove, crushed
1½ tablespoons olive oil
4 boneless, skinless chicken breasts
one 14.5-ounce can diced tomatoes
½ cup vegetable broth
1 tablespoon butter
salt and freshly ground black pepper, to season

* Preheat the broiler. Put the peppers cut side down on a broiler tray, lined with foil if you like. Broil for 15 to 20 minutes until the skin is black and blistered. Meanwhile, cook the onions and garlic gently in 1 tablespoon of the olive oil in a large skillet until soft but not colored.
* Place the chicken breasts between two sheets of plastic wrap and bash with a mallet to flatten to about a ¼-inch thickness. Heat a grill pan, brush with the remaining 1½ teaspoons olive oil, and grill the chicken for about 4 minutes on each side or until cooked through.
* Remove the peppers from the broiler and allow to cool for 5 minutes. When cool enough to handle, remove the skin and chop roughly. Add to the onions with the tomatoes and vegetable broth. Bring to a simmer and add the chicken. Cook for 20 to 25 minutes, turning the chicken halfway through.
* Remove the chicken from the skillet and cut into slices. Stir the sauce until smooth. Stir in the butter and season. Spoon the sauce on top of the chicken and serve with fluffy white rice.

chicken balls in tomato sauce

Meatballs and chicken balls tend to be popular, and this recipe is good made with ground beef, chicken, or turkey. It also freezes well, so it's good to keep some on hand for times when the pantry is bare.

CHICKEN BALLS

2 tablespoons olive oil
1 medium onion, finely chopped
⅓ cup fresh white bread crumbs
(about 2 slices)
¼ cup milk
½ pound ground chicken or turkey
1 small apple, peeled and grated
1 teaspoon chopped fresh thyme
leaves
½ teaspoon salt
freshly ground black pepper,
to season

1 tablespoon all-purpose flour,
to dust hands
3 tablespoons canola oil, for frying

TOMATO SAUCE

1 tablespoon olive oil
1 small red onion, finely chopped
1 garlic clove, crushed
one 14.5-ounce can diced tomatoes
1 tablespoon ketchup
1 teaspoon brown sugar
¼ cup water
salt and freshly ground black
pepper, to season

* To make the chicken balls, heat the 2 tablespoons olive oil in a pan and fry the onion gently for about 10 minutes until softened. Meanwhile, soak the bread crumbs in the milk for 10 minutes in a large bowl.
* Add the chicken or turkey, apple, thyme, sautéed onion, salt, and pepper to the soaked bread crumbs and mix together. Using floured hands, form teaspoonfuls of the mixture into small balls. Heat the canola oil in a frying pan and brown the meatballs. They will be cooked again in the sauce, so cook for only about 5 minutes.
* To make the tomato sauce, heat the 1 tablespoon olive oil and sauté the red onion for 5 minutes. Add the garlic and cook for 1 minute. Add the remaining ingredients. Bring to a simmer and cook for 10 minutes. Add an additional 2 tablespoons water if the sauce thickens too much.
* Add the browned chicken balls to the sauce and cook for about 10 minutes. Serve with rice.

chicken drumsticks with barbecue sauce

Chicken drumsticks with a tasty barbecue sauce are popular with my three children. They can eat two each, but it really depends on how large the drumsticks are. I score the drumsticks a few times to make sure that the meat is cooked all the way through.

6 chicken drumsticks

MARINADE
3 tablespoons ketchup
1 tablespoon canola oil
1 tablespoon rice wine vinegar
1 tablespoon soy sauce
2 tablespoons honey
1 teaspoon paprika
1 garlic clove, crushed

✳ Wash the chicken and pat dry with paper towels. Score each drumstick three times using a sharp knife.
✳ Thoroughly mix together all the ingredients for the marinade. Coat the drumsticks with the marinade and leave to marinate for at least 30 minutes or overnight in the fridge.
✳ Preheat the oven to 400°F. Line a baking sheet or roasting pan with foil. Place the drumsticks on the foil together with the marinade. Roast for 35 to 40 minutes until the chicken is thoroughly cooked.

the one-bowl meal

Some fussy eaters are much happier eating soup. This is a really yummy chicken soup and perfect for when you have leftover roast chicken. With the chicken, rice, and vegetables, it makes a meal in itself.

½ medium onion, chopped
1 tablespoon olive oil
1 medium carrot, diced
2¾ cups good-quality chicken broth
½ teaspoon chopped fresh thyme leaves
½ cup frozen peas
⅔ cup drained canned corn
1 cup shredded cooked chicken
1 cup cooked rice (⅓ cup uncooked)
salt and freshly ground black pepper,
  to season

✳ Sauté the onion gently in the oil for about 5 minutes. Add the carrot, broth, and thyme and simmer for 4 to 5 minutes until the carrot softens. Add the peas and corn and simmer for 3 minutes.
✳ Add the shredded chicken to the soup together with the cooked rice, and simmer for 2 minutes to reheat. Season with a little salt and pepper.

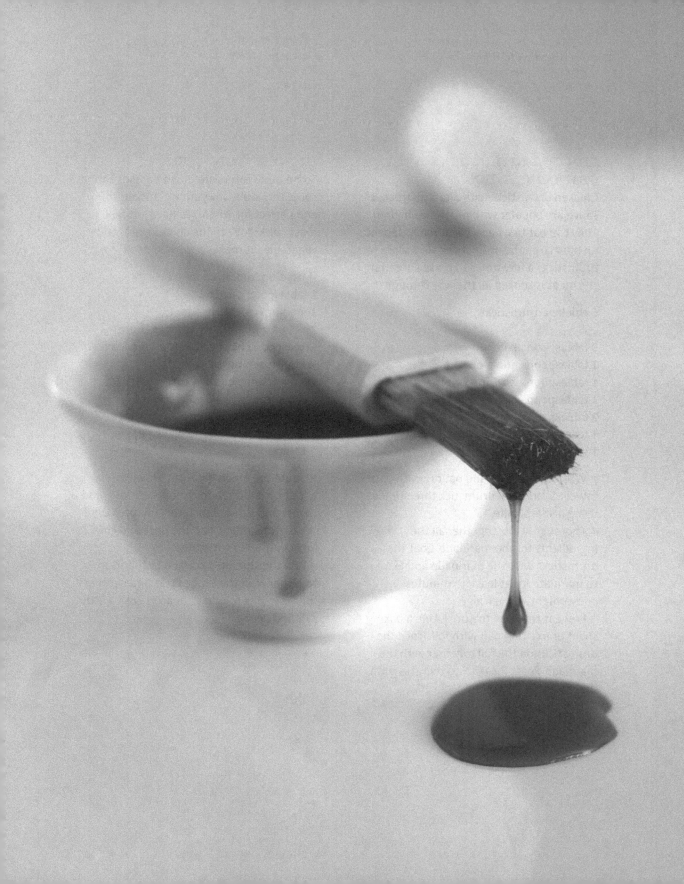

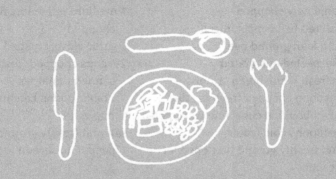

MMM...eat

meatballs with tomato sauce

These mini meatballs are delicious served on a bed of rice. They are simple to prepare and make a wonderful family meal. They also work well as finger food, served on their own without the sauce.

MEATBALLS

1 tablespoon canola oil
1 onion, finely chopped
½ small red bell pepper, diced
1 pound lean ground beef
1 apple, peeled and grated
⅓ cup fresh white bread crumbs
1 tablespoon chopped fresh parsley
1 chicken bouillon cube, finely crumbled
2 tablespoons cold water
salt and freshly ground black pepper,
   to season

all-purpose flour, for dusting
2 tablespoons canola oil

TOMATO SAUCE

1 tablespoon olive oil
1 medium red onion, finely
   chopped
1 garlic clove, crushed
2⅔ cups chopped fresh or
   canned tomatoes
1½ tablespoons ketchup
⅓ cup water
salt and freshly ground black
   pepper, to season

* To make the meatballs, heat the 1 tablespoon canola oil in a pan and sauté the onion and bell pepper for about 5 minutes until softened. Mix together with all the other ingredients for the meatballs and chop for a few seconds in a food processor. Using floured hands, form the mixture into about 20 meatballs. Heat the 2 tablespoons canola oil in a frying pan and sauté the meatballs, turning occasionally, for about 5 minutes, until browned and sealed.
* Meanwhile, to make the sauce, heat the olive oil and sauté the red onion for 5 minutes. Add the garlic and cook for 1 minute. Add the remaining ingredients. Bring to a simmer and cook for 5 minutes. Add a little more water if the sauce thickens too much. Add the meatballs, half cover with a lid, and simmer, stirring occasionally, for about 10 minutes until cooked through. You need to be careful when stirring the meatballs into the sauce, as if you are too vigorous, they may break up. Serve with rice.

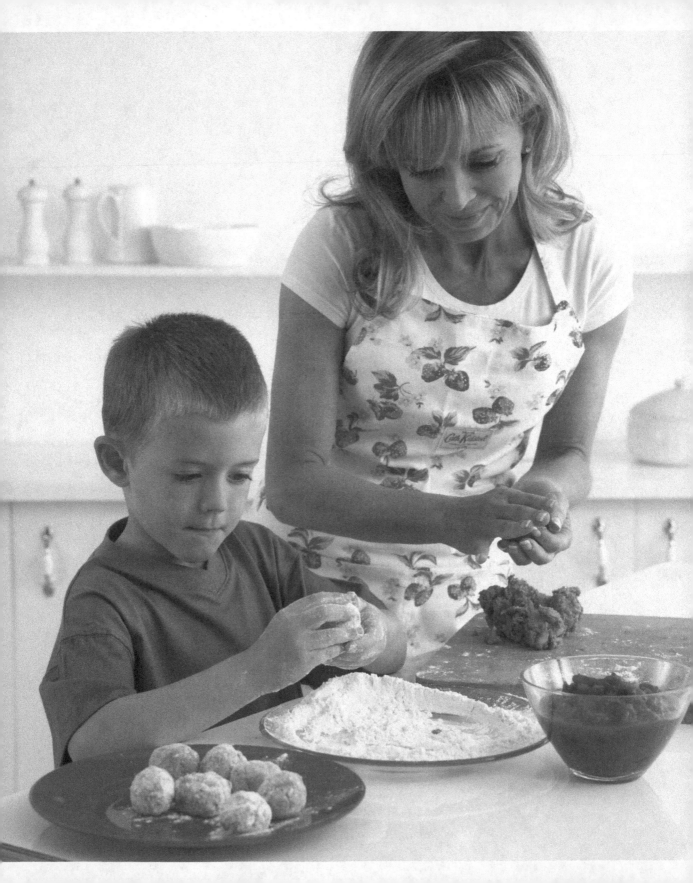

annabel's yummy burgers

Making your own healthy junk food is one way to encourage fussy eaters to eat better-quality food. Adding tomato chutney to burgers gives them a delicious flavor. My children love these. Serve them on their own or in a bun with some lettuce.

1 medium red onion, chopped
3 tablespoons canola oil
1 garlic clove, crushed
½ teaspoon chopped fresh thyme leaves
2 slices white bread, crusts removed
½ pound ground beef
3 tablespoons tomato chutney or tomato relish
salt and freshly ground black pepper, to season
1 to 2 tablespoons all-purpose flour, for dusting

* Sauté the onion in 1 tablespoon of the canola oil for 5 to 6 minutes until soft. Add the garlic and thyme and cook for 1 minute. Tear the bread into pieces and put in a food processor with the onion mixture and blitz.
* If you want a really smooth texture, add the ground beef, chutney, and seasoning to the food processor and pulse for a few seconds. If not, combine with the bread mixture in a bowl. Form the mixture into 4 burgers using flour-dusted hands.
* For the best flavor, I like to cook these on a contact grill that does both sides at once—this method of cooking also halves the cooking time. Alternatively, fry the burgers in the remaining 2 tablespoons oil for 4 to 5 minutes on each side over medium-to-low heat. If you fry over high heat, because of the sugar in the tomato chutney, the burgers have a tendency to burn.

☆ If you want to freeze burgers, it's best to do so uncooked on a tray lined with plastic wrap. When they are frozen, wrap them individually in plastic wrap. You can then use as many as you like.

alison's favorite shepherd's pie

Dr. Alison French is a specialist in pediatrics and child health.
She helps me answer all the e-mails I receive every day via
my Web site. Alison's children, Amelie and Ben, love this recipe.

1½ pounds Yukon Gold or red-skinned potatoes, peeled and cut into chunks
3 tablespoons unsalted butter
6 tablespoons milk
1 tablespoon olive oil
1 large or 2 small onions
2 medium carrots
1 large or 2 small zucchini
½ red bell pepper
1 garlic clove, crushed
1 pound ground lamb (I use organic, as it tastes much better)
1 teaspoon ground cinnamon
1 teaspoon dried mixed herbs, such as Italian seasoning
1 teaspoon superfine sugar
freshly ground black pepper, to season
1 tablespoon all-purpose flour
1 tablespoon tomato paste
1¼ cups hot beef broth
½ cup grated mild Cheddar

* Boil the potatoes until soft and floury (about 15 minutes) and then drain.
Mash with the butter and milk and set aside.
* Heat the olive oil in a large pan. Finely chop the onion, carrot, zucchini, and
bell pepper in a food processor and sauté in the oil for 4 minutes or until soft
but not browned. Add the garlic and cook for 1 minute. Stir in the lamb and turn
up the heat. When the meat is browned, add the cinnamon, herbs, sugar, a little
freshly ground black pepper, and the flour and stir well. Add the tomato paste
to the hot broth and add to the pan. Stir well, and simmer for about 10 minutes.
* Preheat the oven to 350°F. Spoon the meat into a large glass casserole or deep
pie dish. Top the meat mixture with the mashed potatoes and run a fork over it
until it is smooth. Sprinkle the cheese on top and bake in the center of the oven
for about 30 minutes until the top is brown and the meat is bubbling.

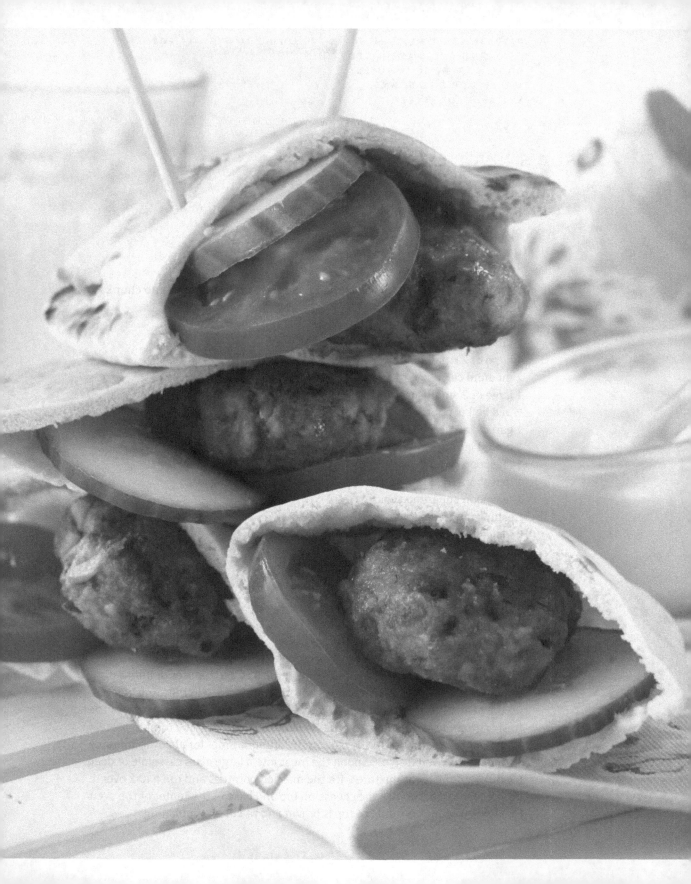

luscious lamb koftas

If your child just won't sit still long enough to eat anything, it might be a good idea to try finger food. Iron is the most common nutritional deficiency in young children, so it's good to make finger foods such as these koftas. Meat provides the best source of iron, which is important for growth and development and crucial in the production of healthy red blood cells, which carry oxygen around the body including to the brain. A deficiency of iron often leads to lack of concentration and tiredness, and ensuring that your child gets enough iron can markedly improve academic performance.

2 onions, chopped
1 tablespoon olive oil
1¼ pounds ground lamb
⅔ cup fresh bread crumbs
2 tablespoons chopped fresh cilantro
2 tablespoons chopped fresh parsley
1 tablespoon mild curry powder
2 teaspoons ground cumin
1 lightly beaten egg
1 beef bouillon cube, crumbled
1 teaspoon sugar
salt and freshly ground black pepper,
   to season
all-purpose flour, for rolling
canola oil, for frying

TO SERVE
7 standard-size pita breads
Greek-style yogurt or other
   thick plain yogurt
14 slices cucumber, preferably
   English or hothouse
14 slices tomato

* Sauté half of the chopped onion in the olive oil until softened. Then mix together the sautéed onion, raw onion, lamb, and all the remaining kofta ingredients (except the flour and vegetable oil). Transfer to a food processor and chop for a few seconds. Form the mixture into 14 koftas (short, fat sausage shapes), roll in flour, and sauté in the canola oil until golden and cooked through.
* Cut the pita pockets in half. Spoon a little yogurt into each pocket and stuff each one with a lamb kofta, a slice of cucumber, and a slice of tomato. If you prefer, serve without the pita pockets and maybe with some couscous or rice instead (as well as the yogurt and salad).

teriyaki beef skewers

The beauty of this is that it is so quick and easy to prepare, and the teriyaki marinade may tempt children who aren't keen on red meat. When grating ginger, grate with the grain—you will see what I mean if you try to do it the other way. Mirin is the key ingredient used to make teriyaki sauce. It is a sweet Japanese rice wine used for cooking. You can buy it in some supermarkets and also Asian food stores.

TERIYAKI SAUCE
1 tablespoon soy sauce
1 tablespoon honey
1 teaspoon mirin
¼ teaspoon grated fresh ginger
1 teaspoon Asian sesame oil
1 teaspoon canola oil

½ pound top loin, shell steak, or other tender steak, fat removed
   and cut into ½-inch cubes
4 bamboo skewers, soaked in water for 20 minues

* To make the teriyaki sauce, put the soy sauce, honey, and mirin in a medium pan. Bring to a boil and cook for 30 seconds (or for 1 minute in a small pan). Allow to cool, then stir in the ginger and oils. Toss the cubed beef in a bowl with the marinade (it will be quite sticky) and marinate for at least 1 hour and preferably overnight in the fridge.
* Preheat the broiler. Remove the meat from the marinade and thread onto the skewers. Place the skewered meat on a baking sheet lined with foil. Baste with some of the marinade left in the bowl and broil for 2 minutes. Turn, baste with the marinade, and broil again for 2 minutes. Baste once more with the marinade and juices collecting in the foil and broil 1 minute longer. Allow to cool slightly before serving. Alternatively, you could cook these on a grill pan.

☆ To make another good teriyaki marinade, put 1 tablespoon soy sauce, 2 tablespoons sake, 2 tablespoons mirin, and 1 tablespoon superfine sugar in a small pan, and heat, stirring, until the sugar has dissolved.

i don't like...

neat that's
not a burger
☹

-takes all Day
to chew

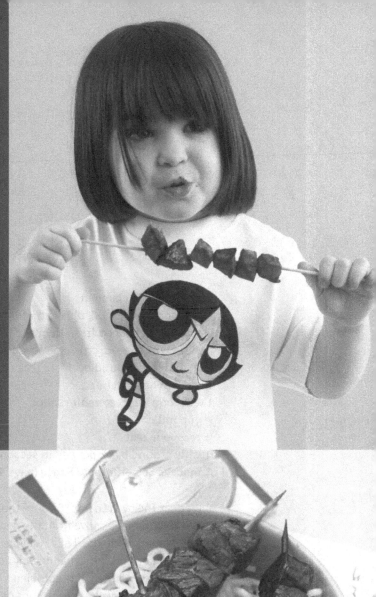

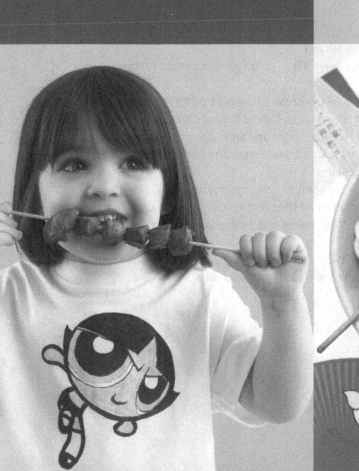

PREPARATION TIME 10 MINUTES
COOKING TIME 15 OR 20 MINUTES
MAKES 6 "REGULAR MUFFINS" OR 12 "MINI MUFFINS"
SUITABLE FOR FREEZING

mini meat loaves

Mini portions are always more attractive to children, so try
making mini meat loaves in a muffin pan. In fact, you can also
make tiny bite-size meat loaves in mini muffin pans.

½ onion, finely chopped
1½ teaspoons olive oil, plus extra for greasing
½ teaspoon chopped fresh thyme
2 slices white bread, crusts removed
½ pound lean ground beef
3 tablespoons ketchup
1 teaspoon Worcestershire sauce
¼ cup milk
½ teaspoon salt
freshly ground black pepper, to season
Annabel's Secret Tomato Sauce (page 45) or your favorite tomato sauce

* Preheat the oven to 400°F. Sauté the onion in the olive oil for 5 minutes, then
stir in the thyme. Remove from the heat and allow to cool slightly. Meanwhile,
put the bread in the bowl of a food processor and whiz into crumbs. Add the
sautéed onion and the remaining ingredients (except the tomato sauce) and
whiz for 1 to 2 minutes until combined.
* Lightly grease 12 mini muffin cups or 6 regular muffin cups. For finger-size
mini meat loaves, put 1 tablespoonful of the meat mixture in each cup of the
mini muffin pan. For the larger meat loaves, put 2 tablespoonfuls in each cup of
the muffin pan.
* Bake for 15 minutes for the mini muffin loaves and 20 minutes for the regular
muffin size. Remove from the pans with a spatula and serve with Annabel's
Secret Tomato Sauce (page 45).

☆ Freeze cooked, preferably in individual portions with some sauce. Thaw
overnight in the fridge or for 1 to 2 hours at room temperature. You can reheat in
a microwave or the oven.

swedish meatballs

2 slices white bread, crusts removed
¼ cup milk
1 large onion, finely chopped
2 tablespoons canola oil
½ pound ground beef
½ pound ground pork
¼ teaspoon grated nutmeg
1 egg yolk
salt and freshly ground black pepper, to season
all-purpose flour, for dusting

SAUCE
1 tablespoon plus 1 teaspoon butter
1 tablespoon plus 1 teaspoon all-purpose flour
1¼ cups good-quality beef broth
⅓ cup heavy cream
salt and freshly ground black pepper, to season

* Preheat the oven to 400°F. Tear the bread into ½-inch pieces and put in a bowl with the milk. Leave to soak for 10 minutes.
* Put the onion in a large saucepan with 1 tablespoon of the oil and sauté for 5 to 6 minutes over medium heat, until the onion is translucent. Transfer roughly two-thirds of the onion to a large bowl and add the milky bread, beef and pork, nutmeg, and egg yolk. Season well with salt and plenty of ground black pepper, then mix until thoroughly combined (for a smoother texture, mix everything in a food processor).
* Put the remaining 1 tablespoon oil on a large baking sheet. Take heaping teaspoons of the meatball mixture and roll into about 25 balls using the palms of your hands—dust your hands with flour to prevent the meatballs from sticking. Put the meatballs on the oiled baking sheet and bake for 20 minutes, turning halfway through.
* Meanwhile, make the sauce. Add the butter to the remaining onion, melt over low heat, and stir in the flour. Cook for 2 minutes, then remove from the heat and stir in the beef stock a little at a time until you have a smooth sauce. Stir in the cream and and cook over medium heat, stirring, for 7 to 8 minutes, until the sauce is just about to boil and has thickened slightly. Season to taste.
* Remove the meatballs from the oven, blot with paper towels, then add the meatballs to the sauce and simmer for 5 minutes before serving.

sticky bbq ribs

These ribs make delicious finger food, and the added attraction
is the sticky mess your child gets into chewing on them, so have
the wet wipes handy.

BBQ SAUCE
1 small red onion, chopped
1 tablespoon olive oil
1 garlic clove, crushed
½ cup ketchup
½ cup fresh orange juice
¼ cup honey
1 tablespoon soy sauce
2 teaspoons Worcestershire sauce

2¾ pounds Saint Louis–style spareribs, cut into individual ribs
salt and freshly ground black pepper, to season

* Preheat the oven to 325°F. In a frying pan, sauté the onion in the oil for
5 minutes or until soft. Add the garlic and cook for 1 minute, then add the
remaining sauce ingredients, bring to a simmer, and cook for 1 minute.
Allow to cool slightly, then whiz together in a blender.
* Put the ribs in a large roasting pan (line with foil for easier cleanup) and
season with salt and pepper. Add the sauce and toss the ribs to coat. Cover with
foil and cook for 30 minutes. Increase the oven temperature to 400°F, uncover
the ribs, and cook for another 30 minutes, turning over halfway through.
Transfer to a plate and allow to cool slightly before serving.
* Alternatively, you can broil or grill the ribs—season and cook in the broiler or
over coals for 10 minutes on each side. Brush the ribs with some of the sauce,
then turn and broil or grill for 5 minutes. Repeat 3 to 4 times until the ribs are
cooked through, with a sticky coating.

☆ You can pop some medium-size baking potatoes into the oven at the same
time as the ribs for a perfect accompaniment. Or boil some corn on the cob
for around 12 minutes, and serve with a little butter.

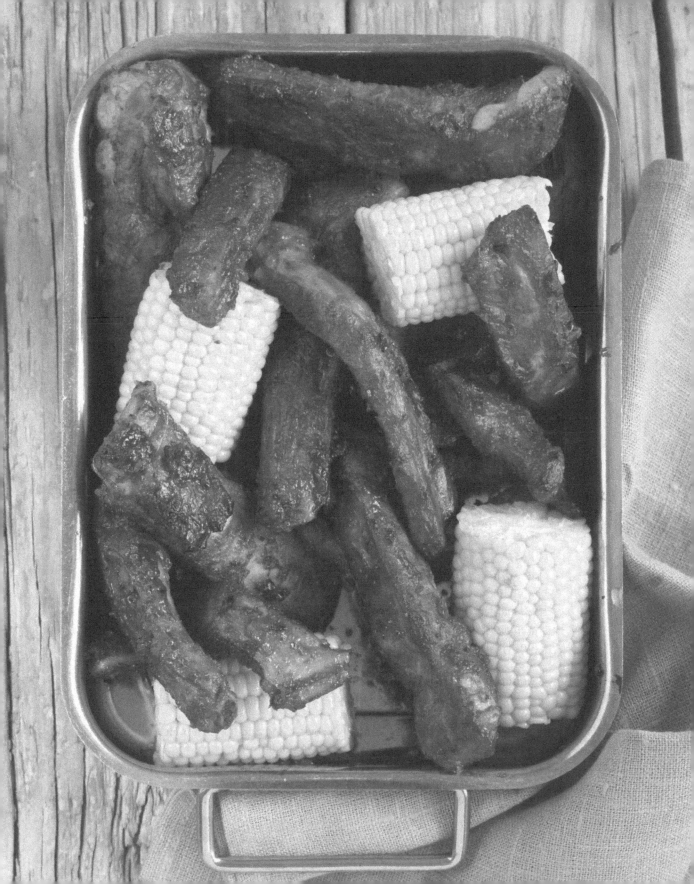

pork medallions with caramelized apples

If your child eats chicken, then he should be tempted by pork, "the other white meat." The sweet caramelized apples will also whet tricky appetites and are a slightly more sophisticated version of applesauce. You could use 4 medium-size boneless pork chops (cook for 6 to 7 minutes each side) instead of the tenderloin if you prefer.

1 pound pork tenderloin, trimmed
1 tablespoon olive oil
salt and freshly ground black pepper, to season
2 tablespoons cider vinegar
½ cup vegetable or chicken broth
2 tablespoons heavy cream

CARAMELIZED APPLES
1 tablespoon butter
1 large eating apple (such as Fuji), peeled, cored, and cut into 12 wedges
1 tablespoon sugar
1 tablespoon water

* To make the medallions, cut the tenderloin into 8 pieces and lay cut side down between 2 pieces of plastic wrap. Tap the pork with a rolling pin into medallions around ½ inch thick.
* Heat the oil in a large frying pan. Season the pork medallions with salt and pepper and fry over medium-high heat for around 3 minutes on each side, until just cooked through (be careful not to overcook, or they will become dry). Transfer to a dish. Add the cider vinegar to the frying pan and boil for 1 minute or until almost evaporated. Add the broth and boil for 2 to 3 minutes, until reduced by half. Stir in the cream, pour the sauce over the pork medallions, and keep warm in a low oven.
* Wipe out the frying pan with paper towels and add the butter. Heat until foaming, then add the apple and cook over medium-high heat for around 2 minutes on each side, until starting to turn golden brown. Sprinkle the sugar and water into the pan and cook, stirring, for another minute or two, until the apples are coated in a thin caramel. Serve with the pork.

lamb lollipops

Frenched lamb chops make great finger food, as they come with their own little "sticks." If the glaze becomes too thick when cool, warm it gently again before brushing on the lamb.

1 tablespoon red currant jelly
1 teaspoon fresh orange juice
a small pinch of ground cinnamon
    (optional)
6 frenched lamb chops
salt and freshly ground black pepper,
    to season

* Preheat the broiler. Put the jelly, orange juice, and cinnamon in a small pan and heat until the jelly has melted. Bring to a boil and cook for around 15 seconds, then set aside to cool and thicken slightly.
* Season the lamb with salt and pepper and broil for 3 to 4 minutes on each side. Allow to cool slightly, then brush with the red currant glaze before serving.

sloppy joe

Sloppy joe is a hot sandwich composed of ground beef seasoned with tomato sauce and served on a bun. The term "sloppy" comes from the fact that the texture is loose. Don't try to pick it up! Serve on a plate. You could also mix this tasty sauce with rice.

1 tablespoon canola oil
½ onion, chopped
1 small carrot, diced
½ celery stalk, diced
⅛ red bell pepper, diced
¾ pound ground beef or turkey
one 14.5-ounce can diced tomatoes,
    with liquid
½ cup chicken broth
2 teaspoons red wine vinegar
2 teaspoons Worcestershire sauce
1 teaspoon brown sugar
1 tablespoon ketchup
a few drops of Tabasco sauce
salt and freshly ground black pepper,
    to season
4 hamburger buns

* Heat the oil in a large frying pan and sauté the vegetables for 5 to 6 minutes. Add the beef or turkey and cook for 3 to 4 minutes until slightly browned. Add all the other ingredients (except the buns) and simmer for 10 minutes. If dry, add an extra ¼ cup chicken broth. Season with salt and pepper. Open each hamburger bun on a plate and spoon the sloppy joe over it.

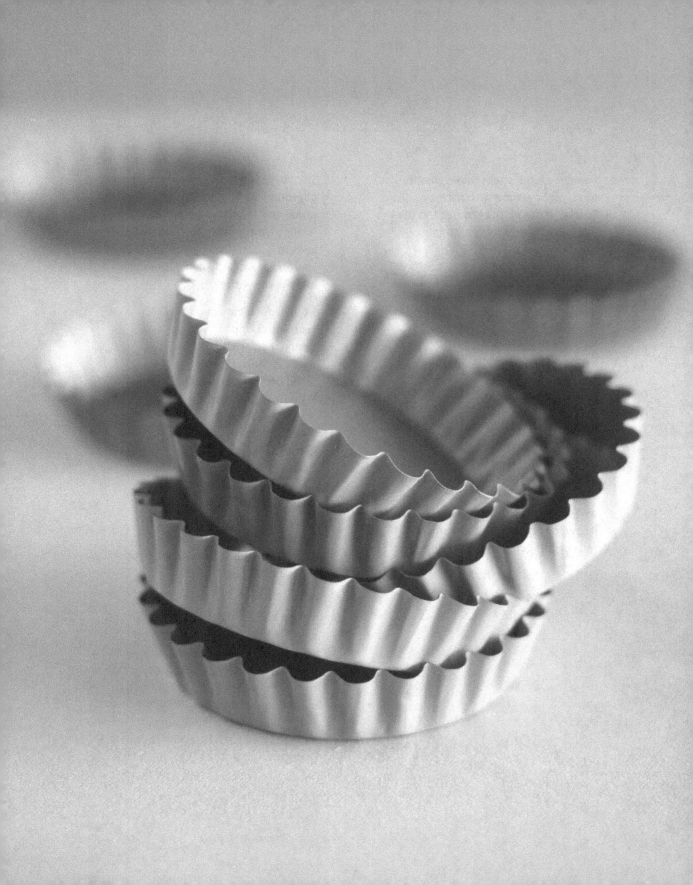

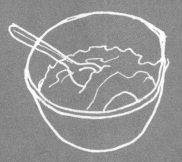

gluten — free
and gorgeous

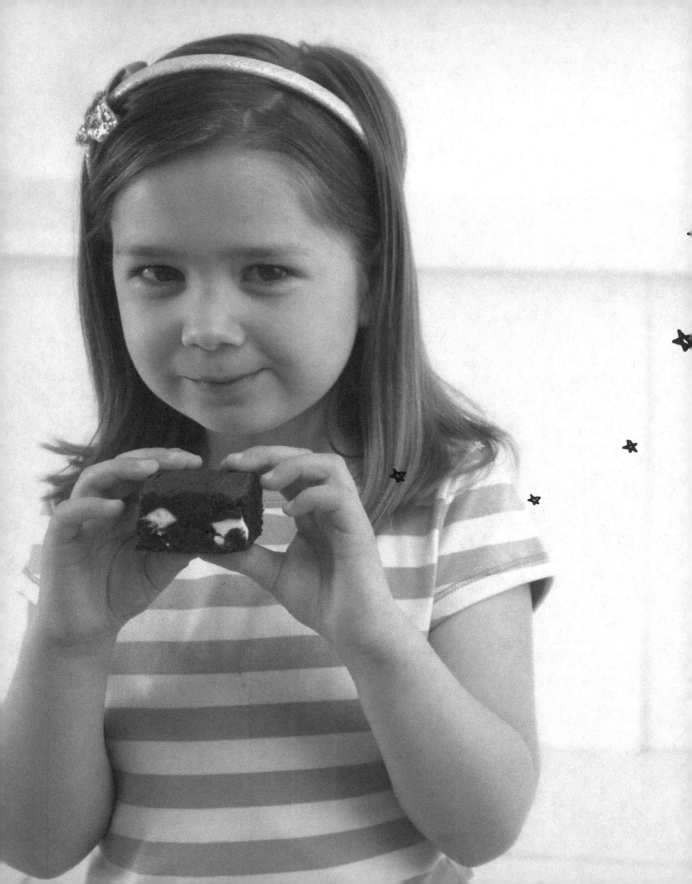

gluten

As food intolerances become more common, I find that many people are looking for recipes that avoid wheat or are suitable for celiacs. It can be a challenge to cook for children who have to avoid wheat or gluten, as they shouldn't feel as if they are missing out on family meals or treats, and it's even more of a struggle if your child is a fussy eater. For this chapter, I have created a collection of recipes that can be enjoyed by the whole family.

While you can buy a good variety of gluten-free foods, many contain additives and preservatives, and more often than not they just don't taste very good. The Celiac Society will provide you with an up-to-date list of gluten-free foods.

Celiac disease used to be considered rare, but now the frequency can be as high as 1 in 100 births. If your child has celiac disease and eats food containing gluten, the gluten damages the lining of the small intestine, which can cause symptoms including vomiting, diarrhea, stomach pains, smelly stools, and a bloated tummy. It also means he or she will have problems absorbing essential nutrients such as calcium and iron. The good news is that as soon as you remove gluten from your child's diet, the symptoms can disappear completely. However, your child will need to follow a gluten-free diet for life—it's not something he or she will grow out of.

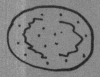

It's important to explain to children why they can't eat certain foods—for example, because those will cause a bad tummy ache—and to make sure there is always an alternative, such as rice noodles instead of wheat pasta. Wheat-free and gluten-free baking can be a pleasure once you have learned to use and feel at home with the ingredients.

* Add slightly more liquid to your recipes because it will be quickly absorbed (and it doesn't mean tough pastry, as there is no gluten).

* You can substitute wheat-free and gluten-free flours for regular flour in many of my recipes, but there are always going to be some that just don't work with gluten-free flour. My advice is that it is generally best to substitute when there is a low ratio of flour to other ingredients, as then you are less reliant on gluten in flour to hold the mixture together.

* Rice flour, polenta, buckwheat flour, and potato flour are fine for celiacs.

* For cakes, make sure you use nonstick pans that are well greased and lined on the bottom for easier turning out— gluten-free baked goods are always, by nature, a little more fragile.

* Many processed foods such as fish sticks and chicken nuggets contain gluten, and some use bread or wheat starch as fillers, so don't give your child any processed foods unless they are labeled gluten-free.

* Corn- or rice-based cereals are fine.

* Crushed cornflakes will make a good coating for chicken nuggets or fish sticks. I have a recipe in the fish chapter for popcorn-coated fish, which is also gluten free if made without the flour (see Crunchy Popcorn Fish, page 83). Crushed plain potato chips are also an option. Or you could use a coating of gluten-free flour, egg, and gluten-free bread crumbs.

* Where a recipe calls for regular flour, mix in 1 teaspoon of gluten-free baking powder to every cup of gluten- or wheat-free flour.

* Where a recipe calls for self-rising flour, mix in 3 to 4 level teaspoons of gluten-free baking powder to every 1½ cups of gluten- or wheat-free flour.

* I find that pastry holds together much better if you mix it with egg rather than just water—the egg helps to act as a binder.

* You may find it easier to roll pastry between two sheets of baking parchment. If you are making lots of gluten-free pastry, it is worth investing in a silicone rolling mat, which makes handling a lot easier.

grace's dairy- and gluten-free bircher muesli

It's a good idea to steer your child away from eating only sugary, refined cereals. Try making your own delicious mueslis—you can customize these by mixing in your child's favorite fruits.

2 cups buckwheat flakes or quick-cooking oats
1½ cups apple juice
2 apples
½ cup chopped sugar-free dried apple
½ cup plain dairy yogurt or soy yogurt
a handful of seasonal berries, such as raspberries and blueberries

* Put the buckwheat flakes or oats in a large mixing bowl and cover with the apple juice. Cover the bowl and leave in the fridge to soak overnight.
* In the morning, peel and grate the apples and add to the buckwheat or oat mixture. Stir in the dried apple and yogurt. Spoon the mixture into bowls. Scatter the berries over each helping and serve immediately.

☆ Alternatively, you could try quinoa flakes, but you will need an extra ½ cup apple juice.

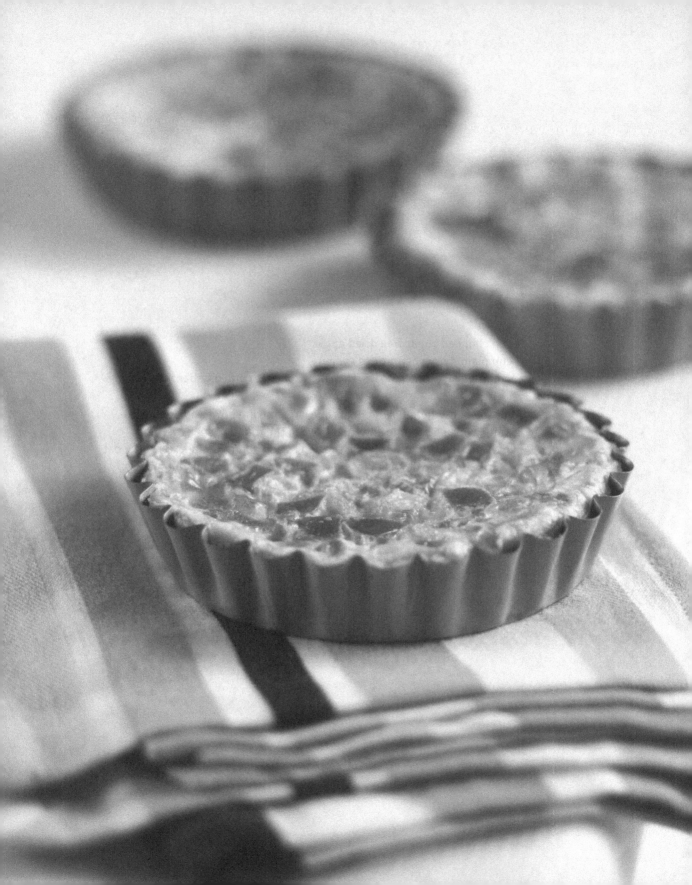

cheesy mini quiches

PASTRY
1 cup rice flour
⅓ cup potato flour
2 teaspoons xanthan gum
½ teaspoon salt
a pinch of cayenne pepper
1 stick cold butter, diced
½ cup grated sharp Cheddar
2 tablespoons freshly grated Parmesan
1 medium egg, lightly beaten

FILLING
3 tablespoons drained canned corn
2 scallions, thinly sliced
1 medium tomato, seeded and diced
½ cup milk
1 medium egg plus 1 egg yolk, lightly beaten
salt and freshly ground black pepper, to season

* To make the pastry, sift together the flours, xanthan gum, salt, and cayenne pepper. Rub in the butter until the mixture looks like sand, then stir in the two cheeses. Add the egg and mix to a dough, adding a few drops of cold water if necessary. (Or pulse the dry ingredients 8 or 9 times in a food processor before adding the egg; then process until a ball of dough forms on the blades.)
* Roll out to ¼-inch thickness and cut out circles using a 3½-inch cutter. Gently lift the circles into the cups of a nonstick muffin pan. Re-roll the trimmings and cut to make a total of 12 quiches. If any cracks appear, then patch with small pieces of pastry. Chill for 30 minutes or until the pastry is firm.
* Preheat the oven to 350°F. Divide the corn, scallions, and tomato among the pastry cases. Put the milk and eggs in a bowl, and whisk to combine thoroughly, then season. Pour the egg mixture into the pastry cases, being careful not to overfill. Bake for 20 to 25 minutes, until the filling is slightly puffed and the pastry is golden. Allow to cool in the pan for 10 minutes.
* Carefully remove the quiches from the pan and allow to cool on a wire rack. Transfer to the fridge as soon as possible if not serving immediately. If cooking from frozen, thaw overnight in the fridge. Warm in a low oven before serving.

chicken and leek pie with potato pastry

You need the mashed potato for this pastry to be fairly dry. To achieve this, it is a good idea to drain the cooked potatoes and allow them to sit in a colander for 10 minutes, or until all of the steam has evaporated, before mashing them without any butter or milk.

FILLING

2 tablespoons butter
1 small onion, chopped
1 medium leek, carefully washed and thinly sliced
1 pound boneless, skinless chicken thighs, cut into ¾-inch cubes
1¾ cups chicken broth
2 tablespoons cornstarch mixed with 2 tablespoons cold water
¼ cup heavy cream
salt and freshly ground black pepper, to season

PASTRY

1½ cups cold mashed potatoes
½ cup cornstarch
½ cup rice flour
½ teaspoon salt
7 tablespoons cold butter, coarsely grated (pop into freezer for 10 minutes
    to make easier to grate)
1 egg, beaten, to glaze

* Melt the butter in a large pan and cook the onion and leek over low heat for around 10 minutes, until translucent. Add the chicken and broth, bring to a simmer, and cook for 6 minutes, then stir in the cornstarch paste and cook for around 2 minutes, until the sauce thickens. Remove from the heat, add the cream, and season to taste with salt and pepper. Transfer to 4 small pie dishes with a lip, or one 8-inch pie plate. Allow to cool, and chill.
* To make the pastry, mix the potato, cornstarch, rice flour, and salt together in a large bowl. Add the butter and work in with your hands, then add up to 2 tablespoons water to mix to a smooth dough. (Or place all the ingredients [except the egg] in a food processor and whiz to a dough.)

* For the small pies, divide the dough into quarters and pat out circles big enough to cover the mini pie dishes. Place the pastry over the pie dishes and seal by crimping the edges with a fork. Chill for 1 hour or until the pastry is firm.

* For the large pie, put the dough onto a piece of plastic wrap and pat or roll out to an 8-inch circle or the same size as the pie plate. Lift the plastic wrap and pastry onto a plate or baking sheet and chill for 1 hour or until firm. Carefully flip the pastry over onto the top of the pie plate (it may help to flip it onto the palm of your hand and then slide it onto the pie plate) and peel off the plastic wrap. Seal the pastry to the pie plate by crimping with a fork or your fingers. Carefully press any cracks together to seal.

* Preheat the oven to 400°F. Brush the top(s) of the pie(s) with the beaten egg and cut a small steam hole in the center using a sharp knife. Bake for 30 minutes (small) or 45 to 50 minutes (large) until the top of the pie is golden and the filling is hot.

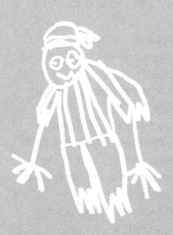

cheesy choux puffs

These small puffs are crisp and cheesy outside, light inside, and delicious served with a tomato dipping sauce.

¼ cup potato flour
½ cup rice flour
½ teaspoon xanthan gum
¼ teaspoon salt
½ cup cold water
4 tablespoons (½ stick) cold butter, cubed
2 medium eggs
½ cup grated Cheddar
1 tablespoon freshly grated Parmesan, plus 1 tablespoon extra for sprinkling (optional)

* Sift together the flours, xanthan gum, and salt twice, and transfer to a piece of baking parchment with a sharp crease in the center. The parchment will help you to form a chute so that you can easily funnel the flour into the pan later.
* Put the water and butter in a medium pan over medium heat. Allow the butter to melt, then bring to a boil for a few seconds. Remove the pan from the heat and funnel the flour into the pan. Immediately beat with a wooden spoon until the mixture forms a ball. Transfer to a large bowl and allow to cool for 10 minutes.
* Beat the eggs into the flour mixture, one at a time, using a wooden spoon, followed by the Cheddar and Parmesan. The choux paste will keep in the fridge for up to 2 days, with plastic wrap pressed on the surface.
* Preheat the oven to 400°F. Spoon the choux paste onto lightly oiled baking sheets, and sprinkle with the extra Parmesan (if using).
* Bake without opening the oven door for the first 20 minutes. Small puffs should be firm and browned on the outside after 20 minutes. Large puffs need 25 minutes. Remove from the oven and cut in half. Scoop out the soft centers and discard and return the shells to the oven for another 5 minutes, until crisp. To serve as rolls, bake for 30 minutes and retain the centers.
* Store in an airtight container for 1 day, or freeze; thaw at room temperature for around 2 hours. Reheat in a 400°F oven for 5 to 10 minutes.

PREPARATION TIME 10 MINUTES
COOKING TIME 15 MINUTES
MAKES 18 TO 20 COOKIES
SUITABLE FOR FREEZING

flourless peanut butter and chocolate chip cookies

Peanut butter with chocolate is always a winning combination for fussy eaters. These cookies taste so good that your child will never know they are made without flour.

1 cup smooth peanut butter, at room temperature
¾ cup superfine sugar
1 medium egg
¼ teaspoon baking soda
a large pinch of salt
¾ cup milk chocolate chips or chopped milk chocolate

* Preheat the oven to 350°F.
* Put the peanut butter, sugar, egg, baking soda, and salt in a large bowl and mix with a wooden spoon until thoroughly combined. Mix in the chocolate chips.
* Take rounded tablespoons of the mixture and roll into balls. It helps to dip the spoon in water every couple of cookies. Put the balls on baking sheets, spaced 2 inches apart. Flatten the balls slightly with your fingers and bake for 12 to 15 minutes. The cookies should have spread out to around ¼ inch thick and have a slightly cracked surface.
* Allow the cookies to cool on the baking sheets for 10 minutes before carefully transferring to wire racks, using a spatula. Allow to cool thoroughly and store in an airtight container for up to 3 days or freeze. If frozen, thaw by spreading out on a baking sheet or plate and leave at room temperature for 30 minutes.

polenta mini pizzas

Polenta is golden-yellow cornmeal made from ground corn. The instant or quick-cooking variety can be made in minutes, and if you flavor it with vegetable broth and Parmesan, it tastes delicious. Cut into circles, it makes a good base for pizzas. Leftover polenta can be cut into squares or triangles and baked as a side dish, or coated in gluten-free flour mixed with Parmesan and fried.

BASE
3¼ cups vegetable broth
1¼ cups instant polenta
¾ to 1 cup freshly grated Parmesan
salt and freshly ground black pepper, to season

TOPPING
¼ cup Annabel's Secret Tomato Sauce (page 45) or store-bought pasta sauce
½ cup grated Cheddar or mozzarella
toppings of your choice, such as strips of ham, bell pepper, and tomato

* Bring the vegetable broth to a boil in a large saucepan and pour in the polenta in a thin stream, whisking constantly. Cook, stirring, until the polenta is thick, 3 to 5 minutes. Remove from the heat and stir in the Parmesan and salt and pepper to taste. Spread the polenta out on a lightly oiled baking sheet to around ¼-inch thickness. Allow to cool, then chill until set—around 1 hour.
* Preheat the oven to 400°F. Cut out 4 large circles using a 3½-inch cutter. (Alternatively, cut the base into a pretty shape, like the flower-shaped one in the photograph.) Top each pizza with 1 tablespoonful of sauce and some grated cheese. Add any other toppings that you like. Transfer the pizzas to a lightly oiled baking sheet and bake for 13 to 15 minutes, until the cheese is bubbling.
* You can freeze these pizzas already assembled and bake from frozen, adding 2 to 3 minutes to the baking time.

polenta mini pizzas

TOPPINGS
Another good topping for the polenta base is caramelized red onion, flavored with balsamic vinegar and thyme and then topped with melted cheese.

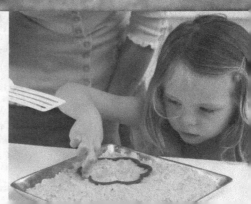

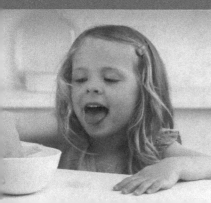
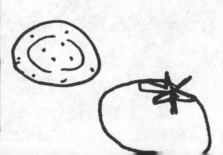

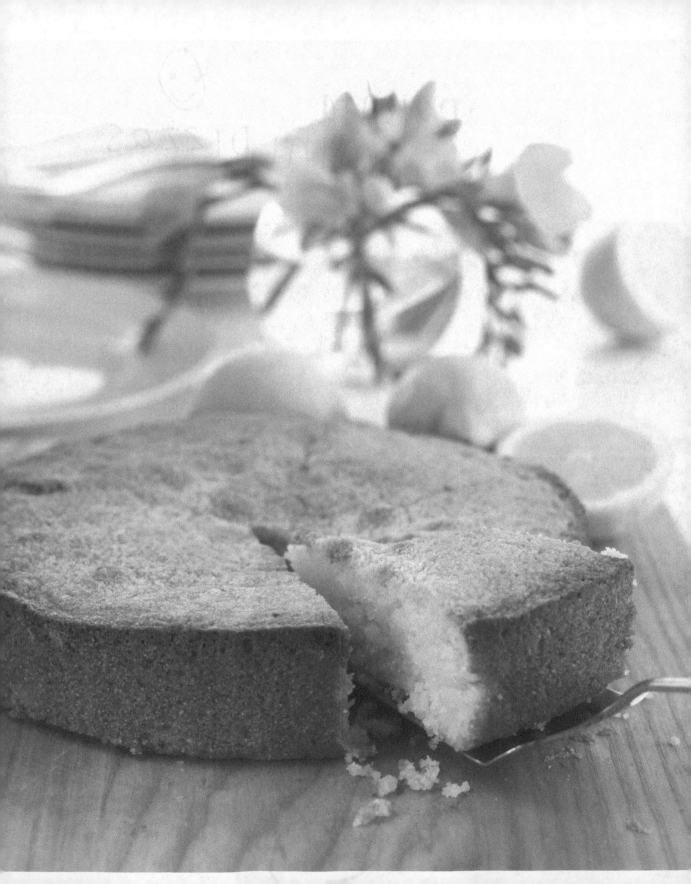

the perfect lemon polenta cake

It can be hard to find a truly delicious cake that doesn't contain any flour. Yes, you can buy gluten-free cakes, but sadly I find them disappointing. When it came to writing this chapter, there was one cake I just had to include, and so I rang Ruth Rogers and Rose Gray of the River Café to see if I could include their wonderful polenta cake—this recipe comes from the original *River Café Cookbook*. I am sure many children, regardless of whether they suffer a wheat allergy or not, will be very grateful.

gluten-free all-purpose flour, to dust
1 pound unsalted butter, softened
1 pound superfine sugar
1 pound almond flour
2 teaspoons vanilla extract
6 eggs
grated zest of 4 lemons
juice of 1 lemon
1½ cups polenta
1 teaspoon gluten-free baking powder
½ teaspoon salt

* Preheat the oven to 300°F. Butter and flour a 12-inch round cake pan.
* Using an electric mixer, beat the butter and sugar together until pale and light. Stir in the almond flour and vanilla. Beat in the eggs, one at a time. Fold in the lemon zest and juice, polenta, baking powder, and salt.
* Spoon into the prepared pan and bake for 45 to 50 minutes until set. The cake will be brown on top. Serve on its own or with ice cream.

gluten-free brownies

These gooey, chewy brownies are so good that you will love them whether you have a gluten allergy or not. You can replace half of the white chocolate with roughly chopped pecans. These are also excellent served as a dessert with vanilla ice cream.

7 ounces semisweet chocolate, cut into chunks
1¾ sticks butter, cut into ½-inch chunks
3 large eggs
1 cup packed light brown sugar
1 cup gluten-free all-purpose flour
3 tablespoons unsweetened cocoa powder
2 teaspoons gluten-free baking powder
a large pinch of salt
6 ounces white chocolate, chopped into chunks
confectioners' sugar, to dust (optional)

* Preheat the oven to 300°F. Put the semisweet chocolate and butter in a heatproof bowl over a pan of simmering water and stir until melted. Alternatively, put the chocolate and butter in a suitable bowl, microwave for 1 minute, stir, then microwave in 10-second blasts until melted. Allow to cool slightly.
* Using an electric mixer, whisk the eggs and light brown sugar together until just combined. Stir in the chocolate and then sift and fold in the flour, cocoa powder, baking powder, and a large pinch of salt. Fold in the white-chocolate chunks.
* Line an 11 x 7-inch cake pan with baking parchment, with the parchment coming up the sides of the pan. Pour the mixture into the pan and bake for 30 minutes or until a crust has formed on the top but there is some give underneath when pressed. Do not overbake. Remove from the oven and allow to cool thoroughly in the pan—don't worry, it will sink and crack a little.
* Remove from the pan and cut into squares before serving. You can dust with confectioners' sugar if you wish.

i don't like...

anything
without chocolate
☹

— what's the point?

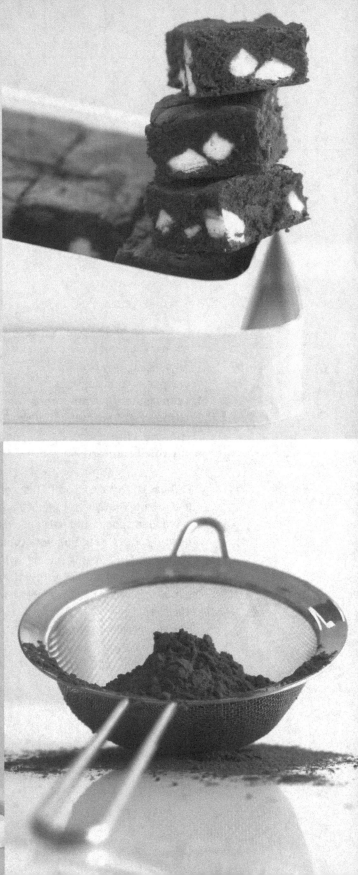

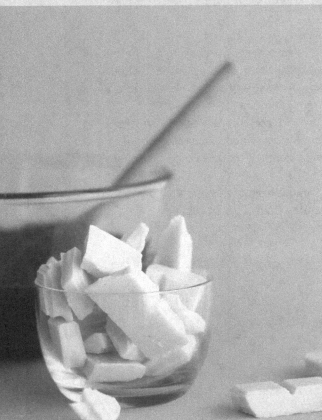

cranberry and white chocolate cookies

You can't compare store-bought cookies to homemade cookies. This combination of cranberry and white chocolate is a real winner. I tend not to add nuts when making cookies for fussy children, because a lot of children refuse to eat anything with nuts in it, but for adults it's good to add ⅔ cup chopped pecans.

1 stick plus 1 tablespoon lightly salted butter, softened
1 cup packed light brown sugar
1 large egg, lightly beaten
½ teaspoon vanilla extract
1⅓ cups gluten-free all-purpose flour, sifted
1 teaspoon gluten-free baking powder
3½ ounces white chocolate, chopped into chunks (⅔ cup)
½ cup dried cranberries

* Preheat the oven to 400°F. Line 2 or 3 baking sheets with baking parchment.
* In a mixing bowl, beat the butter and sugar together using an electric mixer or a wooden spoon until pale and creamy. Add the egg and vanilla a little at a time and continue beating until thoroughly combined.
* Stir in the flour, baking powder, white chocolate, cranberries, and 1½ to 2 tablespoons water and mix until thoroughly combined. Place tablespoons of the mixture on the baking sheets, leaving plenty of space, as they will spread in the oven.
* Bake for 15 minutes or until golden. Remove from the oven and allow to cool on the baking sheets for 2 to 3 minutes, then place on cooling racks.
* Store in an airtight container.

☆ The mixture is quite soft when you spoon it onto the baking sheets, and the cookies are soft when they first come out of the oven, but when they cool down, they will harden. This is a good recipe for children to make with you, as it's so quick and easy to prepare.

blueberry muffins

Blueberries are enjoyed by many children, and these blueberry muffins are popular at breakfast or as a snack. The sour cream makes them nice and moist.

2¼ cups gluten-free all-purpose flour
a large pinch of salt
1 tablespoon gluten-free baking powder
scant 1 cup superfine sugar
1 cup blueberries
2 large eggs
⅔ cup canola oil
⅔ cup sour cream
1 teaspoon vanilla extract
juice and grated zest of 1 small lemon

* Preheat the oven to 375°F. Line a muffin pan with 12 paper cases.
* Stir together the flour, salt, baking powder, sugar, and blueberries. Whisk together the eggs, oil, sour cream, vanilla, and lemon juice and zest (it will look a bit curdled). Stir the wet ingredients into the dry ingredients and spoon into the muffin cases until about three-quarters full.
* Bake for 20 to 25 minutes. Allow to cool in the pan for 5 minutes before removing. Best served warm, though you can store them for a day in an airtight container or freeze.

☆ A bowl of blueberries makes a good snack. According to researchers at Boston University, they top the list in terms of antioxidant activity when compared with forty other fresh fruits and vegetables. While they contain well-known antioxidants such as vitamins C and E, their main health benefits come from the pigment (anthocyanin) that gives blueberries their blue color.

wheat-free birthday cake

Children with celiac disease can feel particularly left out at birthdays without a cake and candles. You can fill this one with jam and vanilla buttercream or use the chocolate buttercream.

2⅔ cups gluten-free all-purpose flour
a large pinch of salt
1 tablespoon gluten-free baking powder
1 stick plus 2 tablespoons unsalted butter, melted
¾ cup milk
¾ cup canola oil
1¼ cups superfine sugar
4 medium eggs
2 teaspoons vanilla extract

VANILLA BUTTERCREAM
1 stick unsalted butter, softened
1⅓ cups confectioners' sugar
½ teaspoon vanilla extract
1 tablespoon milk

4 to 5 tablespoons raspberry jam, for spreading
1½ tablespoons confectioners' sugar, to dust

CHOCOLATE BUTTERCREAM
2 ounces semisweet chocolate
1 stick unsalted butter, softened
1¼ cups confectioners' sugar
1 tablespoon milk

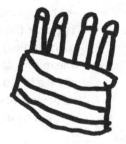

* Preheat the oven to 350°F. Grease two 8-inch round baking pans and line with waxed paper. Sift together the flour, salt, and baking powder. Mix together the melted butter, milk, and oil.
* Whisk the superfine sugar, eggs, and vanilla together until pale and frothy. Whisk in one-third of the oil-and-milk mixture followed by one-third of the sifted flour. Repeat twice. Pour into the cake pans (the mixture will be very liquid). As the mixture is so liquid, you may want to put a baking sheet on the rack underneath the pans to catch any drips.

* Bake for 40 to 45 minutes, until a skewer inserted into the center comes out clean. Allow to cool for 10 minutes in the pans, then turn out the cakes. Allow to cool thoroughly on a wire rack and peel off the lining paper.

* To make the vanilla buttercream, beat the butter until pale and fluffy and beat in the confectioners' sugar a little at a time. Beat in the vanilla and the milk a teaspoonful at a time until the buttercream is spreadable (you may not need all the milk). Spread the jam on top of one of the cake layers and then spread with the buttercream. Cover this with the other cake layer and dust with confectioners' sugar.

* To make the chocolate buttercream, first break the chocolate into pieces and melt in a heatproof bowl over a pan of simmering water. Alternatively, melt in a suitable bowl in a microwave. Allow to cool down a little. Beat the butter until pale and fluffy and beat in the confectioners' sugar a little at a time. Fold in the melted chocolate followed by the milk.

PREPARATION TIME 15 MINUTES
COOKING TIME 25 MINUTES
MAKES 8 CUPCAKES
SUITABLE FOR FREEZING (UN-ICED)

vanilla cupcakes

It's just no fun if you go to a birthday party and can't eat any of the cake, so here's a recipe that doesn't contain gluten but produces deliciously light little cupcakes.

1 stick unsalted butter, softened
½ cup superfine sugar
2 large eggs, at room temperature
½ cup gluten-free all-purpose flour
½ cup almond flour
1 teaspoon gluten-free baking powder
a pinch of salt
1 teaspoon vanilla extract

* Preheat the oven to 350°F. Line a muffin pan with 8 paper cases.

* Beat the butter and sugar until pale and fluffy. Add the remaining ingredients and mix to combine.

* Spoon into the paper cases and bake for 20 to 25 minutes, until risen and firm to the touch. Allow to cool for 5 minutes in the pan, then transfer to a rack until completely cooled.

* You can ice these with buttercream (see birthday cake recipe, opposite) or glacé icing made from confectioners' sugar and a little warm water. Store in an airtight container for up to 5 days or freeze (un-iced).

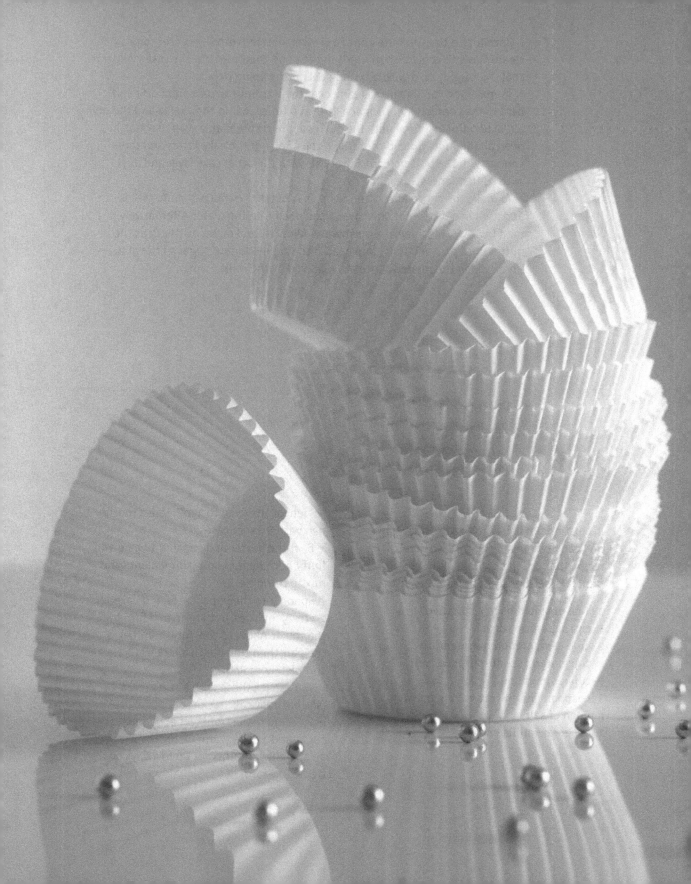

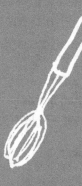

Cookies and cakes

trail mix bars

Trail mix is a snack food commonly used in outdoor recreational activities such as hiking, backpacking, and mountaineering. It usually consists of a mixture of nuts, seeds, and dried fruits such as raisins and cranberries. It's energy rich and has a high content of vitamins and minerals. Fussy eaters often eat more between meals than they do at mealtimes, so it's important to give them healthy snacks such as these bars rather than letting them graze on empty calories that will spoil their appetite for their main meal.

4 tablespoons (½ stick) unsalted butter
3 tablespoons golden syrup, such as Lyle's, or honey
1⅓ cups quick-cooking oats
½ cup packed light brown sugar
¾ cup Cheerios
¼ cup raisins
2 tablespoons salted peanuts or pumpkin seeds
¼ cup milk chocolate chips or dried cranberries
¼ cup sunflower seeds
¼ teaspoon salt

* Preheat the oven to 325°F. Line an 8-inch square pan with baking parchment and grease lightly.
* Put the butter and golden syrup in a small pan over low heat until the butter has melted. Set aside to cool.
* Put the remaining ingredients in a large bowl and stir together. Add the cooled butter mixture and mix well to combine. Transfer the mixture to the prepared pan and press down firmly. Bake for 30 to 35 minutes until the center is just firm to the touch.
* Remove from the oven, allow to cool for 15 minutes, then cut into 8 bars, using a sharp knife. Allow to cool completely before lifting from the pan. Store in an airtight container.

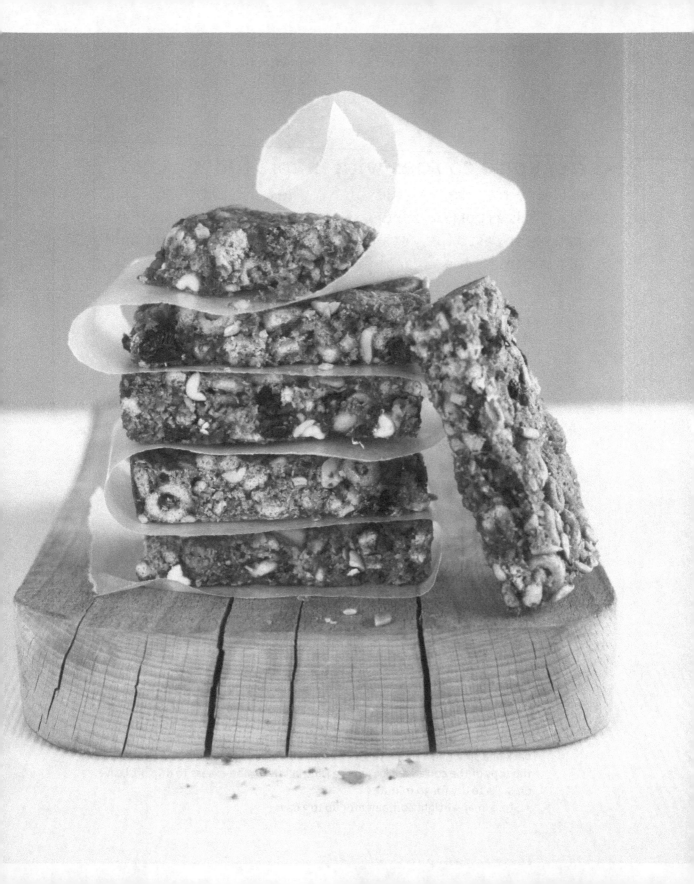

carrot spice cookies with maple fudge glaze

If you love carrot cake, then this is the cookie for you. With oats and carrots, this is a cookie with at least a few healthy ingredients that you can sneak past a fussy eater. If you make these cookies without the glaze, increase the sugar to ½ cup.

1 stick unsalted butter, melted and cooled
⅓ cup superfine sugar
1 egg yolk
⅔ cup all-purpose flour
1½ teaspoons pumpkin pie spice
½ teaspoon salt
1 cup quick-cooking oats
2 medium carrots, grated
⅓ cup raisins

MAPLE FUDGE GLAZE
⅔ cup confectioners' sugar
1 tablespoon unsalted butter, melted
3 tablespoons maple syrup
2 to 4 tablespoons milk

* Preheat the oven to 350°F. Line 3 large baking sheets with baking parchment.
* In a large bowl, mix together the butter, sugar, and egg yolk. In another large bowl, combine the flour, pumpkin pie spice, salt, oats, carrots, and raisins. Add to the butter and stir until well combined.
* Take tablespoons of the dough and roll into walnut-size balls. Put on the baking sheets and flatten slightly to ¾ inch thick. Bake for 20 to 25 minutes until golden, rotating the baking sheets halfway through. Allow to cool on wire racks.
* To make the glaze, mix together the confectioners' sugar, melted butter, maple syrup, and 2 tablespoons milk. If the glaze is too thick (it should coat the back of a spoon in a thin layer), then add more milk, a teaspoon at a time. Dip the tops of the cooled cookies in the icing, allowing the excess to drip off. Leave on racks to dry for 30 minutes.
* Store in an airtight container for up to 3 days.

carrot bar cake

Big portions can be off-putting for fussy eaters, so I have opted to turn the traditional round carrot cake into a bar cake that is more suitable for cutting into kid-friendly squares.

1⅔ cups all-purpose flour
2 teaspoons baking powder
¼ teaspoon baking soda
1 teaspoon ground cinnamon
1 teaspoon ground ginger
½ teaspoon salt
half an 8-ounce can pineapple
   chunks or rings, drained
3 medium carrots, grated
⅔ cup superfine sugar
½ cup canola oil
3 large eggs
½ cup raisins (optional)

CREAM CHEESE ICING
6 ounces cream cheese, at room
   temperature
1 stick unsalted butter, softened
⅓ cup confectioners' sugar
2 tablespoons maple syrup

* Preheat the oven to 350°F. Line an 11 × 7-inch cake pan with baking parchment and grease with a little oil.
* Put all the cake ingredients (except for the raisins) in a food processor. Whiz for 1 to 1½ minutes to make a batter. At this point, you can stir in the raisins, if using.
* Bake for 30 to 35 minutes until firm to the touch and a skewer inserted in the center of the cake comes out clean. Allow to cool in the pan for 15 minutes, then turn out onto a wire rack and allow to cool thoroughly before icing.
* When it comes to icing the cake, it is important that everything be at room temperature, otherwise the butter and cream cheese won't blend properly. Beat together the butter and cream cheese until smooth. Beat in the confectioners' sugar and maple syrup and spread over the cake. Cut into squares before serving.

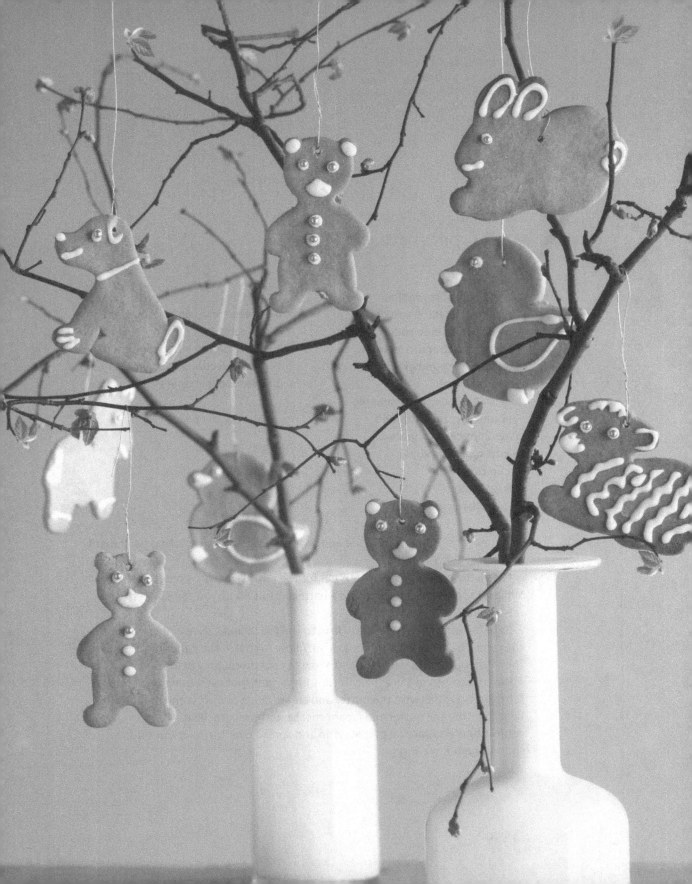

my favorite gingersnaps

These delicious, slightly chewy gingersnaps are great fun to make, as children love rolling out dough and cutting it into shapes using cookie cutters.

5 tablespoons unsalted butter, softened
⅓ cup packed light brown sugar
¼ cup golden syrup, such as Lyle's, or light corn syrup
1¼ cups all-purpose flour, sifted
1 teaspoon ground ginger
½ teaspoon baking soda
a tube of white icing

* Preheat the oven to 350°F.
* Beat the butter and sugar with an electric mixer until pale. Add the golden syrup, flour, ginger, and baking soda and beat together until you form a dough. Wrap in plastic wrap and chill for at least 30 minutes.
* Roll out on a floured work surface to a thickness of about ¼ inch. Start in the center of the dough and roll evenly outward. Cut into shapes using cookie cutters, working from the outside edges of the dough into the center, cutting as close together as possible. Re-roll the trimmings until all the dough is used up.
* Place on baking sheets lined with baking parchment and bake for about 8 minutes. Allow to cool for a few minutes, then transfer to wire racks to cool completely.
* Decorate using the tube of white icing.

my favorite gingersnaps

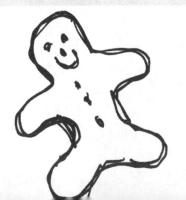

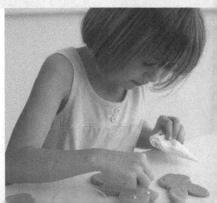

jamaican banana muffins

The smell of these baking should lure many children into the kitchen, eager for the crisp cinnamon crust and moist banana muffin underneath. For maximum flavor, make sure that you use very ripe bananas.

⅓ cup canola oil
½ cup packed light brown sugar
2 medium very ripe bananas, mashed
1 medium egg
1 heaping cup all-purpose flour
2 tablespoons whole wheat flour, sifted
½ teaspoon salt
½ teaspoon baking soda
1½ teaspoons ground cinnamon
3 tablespoons very hot water
½ cup raisins

TOPPING
1 teaspoon ground cinnamon
⅓ cup granulated sugar
1 tablespoon butter, melted

* Preheat the oven to 350°F. Line a muffin pan with 8 paper cases.
* Mix together the oil and sugar. Add the mashed bananas and mix thoroughly. Beat the egg with a fork, add to the banana mixture, and mix well.
* Sift the flours, salt, baking soda, and ground cinnamon into a medium bowl. Add the little bits that were sifted out of the whole wheat flour. Add half the flour mixture to the banana mixture and mix well. Add the hot water and mix in thoroughly. Mix in the remaining flour and the raisins.
* Divide the mixture among the muffin cases.
* Combine the topping ingredients in a small bowl and sprinkle evenly over the muffins. Bake for 25 to 30 minutes until the muffins are well risen and spring back gently when you press the tops. Transfer to a wire rack to cool.

☆ For a gluten-free version, use ⅓ cup canola oil, 1⅓ cups gluten-free all-purpose flour, 1 teaspoon baking soda, and 2 tablespoons hot milk instead of water. Bake for 30 to 35 minutes.,

yogurt "pot" cupcakes

Children will love helping to make this recipe, as much of the measuring is done with one yogurt container, or "pot."

one 6-ounce container plain whole-milk yogurt
two 6-ounce yogurt containers all-purpose flour
1½ teaspoons baking powder
a pinch of salt
1 extra-large egg, lightly beaten
1 yogurt container superfine sugar
¾ yogurt container canola oil
¾ yogurt container chopped dried apricots
1 teaspoon vanilla extract
¼ cup flaked unsweetened coconut

APRICOT BUTTERCREAM
1 tablespoon apricot glaze or 3 tablespoons apricot jam plus
   1 tablespoon water
1 stick plus 2 tablespoons butter, softened
a few drops of vanilla extract
¼ cup confectioners' sugar

edible sugar flowers, to decorate (optional)

* Preheat the oven to 350°F. Line a muffin pan with 12 paper cases.
* Scoop the yogurt out of the container into a large bowl. Rinse out the container and dry it well. Use the container to measure the flour and put this in a separate bowl with the baking powder and salt.
* Add the beaten egg to the yogurt, along with the sugar, then measure and add the oil. Stir in the chopped apricots. Stir in the vanilla, followed by the flour mixture. Finally fold in the coconut. Spoon the batter into the paper cases and bake for about 20 minutes, until risen, golden, and firm to the touch. Allow to cool for 10 minutes in the pan, then transfer to a wire rack to cool completely.
* To make the buttercream, beat together the apricot glaze, butter, and the vanilla, then beat in the confectioners' sugar. If you can't find apricot glaze, heat 3 tablespoons of apricot jam in a saucepan together with 1 tablespoon of water, strain, and allow to cool before use.
* Ice the top of each cupcake, and decorate with an edible sugar flower, if you like. Store in an airtight container for up to 5 days.

oat, apple, and sunflower seed muffins

Muffins make a good snack, as you can sneak in healthy ingredients, and they make good portable food.

2¼ cups all-purpose flour

¾ cup packed light brown sugar

2 teaspoons baking powder

½ teaspoon salt

1 teaspoon ground ginger

½ teaspoon pumpkin pie spice

½ cup quick-cooking oats

2 medium eating apples, peeled, cored, and chopped into small dice

¼ cup sunflower seeds

¼ cup raisins

½ cup canola oil

¼ cup golden syrup, such as Lyle's, or light corn syrup

2 medium eggs, lightly beaten

¾ cup milk

TOPPING

2 tablespoons quick-cooking oats

2 tablespoons sunflower seeds

2 tablespoons turbinado sugar or granulated sugar

* Preheat the oven to 400°F. Line a muffin pan with 12 paper cases.
* Sift the flour, sugar, baking powder, salt, ginger, and pumpkin pie spice into a large bowl, rubbing any lumps of sugar through the sieve. Stir in the oats, apples, sunflower seeds, and raisins.
* Whisk together the oil, syrup, eggs, and milk until thoroughly combined, then stir into the dry ingredients. Spoon into the muffin cases.
* Stir together the topping ingredients and divide among the muffins. Bake for 20 to 22 minutes, until risen and firm to the touch. Allow to cool in the pan, then transfer to a wire rack to cool completely. Keep in an airtight container for up to 3 days.

PREPARATION TIME 15 MINUTES
COOKING TIME 20 MINUTES
MAKES 8 PORTIONS
SUITABLE FOR FREEZING

chocolate pudding cakes with chocolate fudge sauce

Always a favorite in my house. Even the fussiest of eaters wouldn't say no to this!

CHOCOLATE SPONGE

1 stick unsalted butter, softened, plus 1 tablespoon extra for greasing

¾ cup packed light brown sugar

3 large eggs, lightly beaten

¾ cup all-purpose flour

¼ cup unsweetened cocoa powder

2 teaspoons baking powder

¼ teaspoon salt

3 ounces semisweet chocolate, chopped

CHOCOLATE FUDGE SAUCE

4 ounces semisweet chocolate, chopped

¼ cup packed light brown sugar

2 tablespoons golden syrup, such as Lyle's, or light corn syrup

2 tablespoons unsalted butter

1 cup heavy cream

vanilla ice cream, to serve

* Preheat the oven to 350°F. Grease 8 cups of a jumbo muffin pan and line the bottoms with circles of baking parchment.

* Cream the butter and sugar until fluffy. Add the eggs and sift the flour, cocoa, baking powder, and salt into the mixture and beat until just combined. Fold in the chopped chocolate.

* Spoon the batter into the prepared muffin cups (to half full). Bake for 20 minutes or until risen and firm to the touch. Allow to cool slightly, then turn out the pudding cakes (you may need to run a knife around the edges).

* To make the fudge sauce, put all of the ingredients in a medium pan and heat gently until smooth. Bring to a boil, then remove from the heat and pour over the warm cakes. Serve with vanilla ice cream.

☆ You could also bake the chocolate sponge in an 8-inch square cake pan lined with parchment. Baking time may be a bit longer (30 to 35 minutes). Cut into squares and serve with the chocolate sauce.

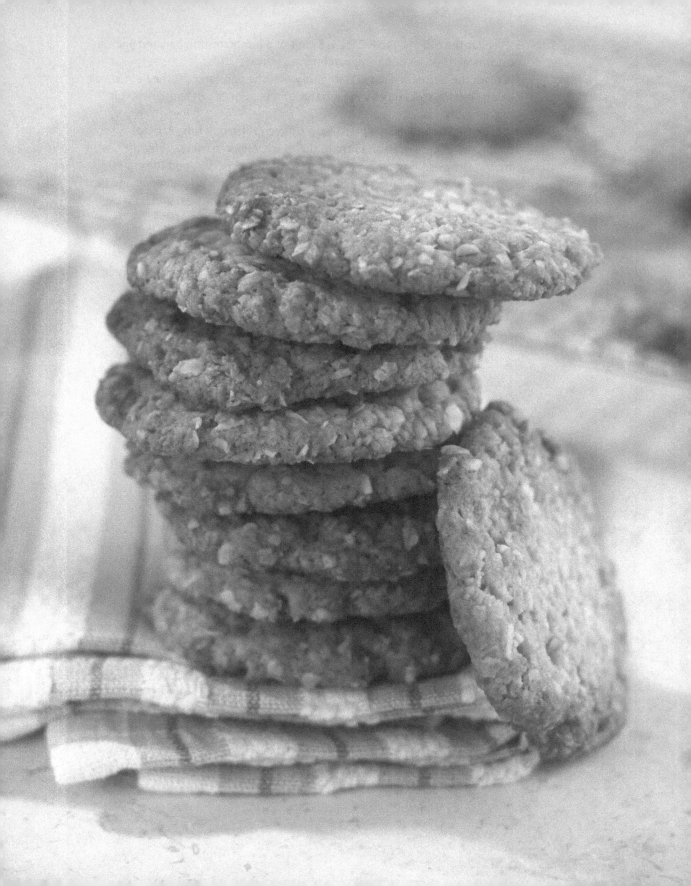

anzac cookies

There are a few theories on the origins of Anzac cookies, but it is certain that they were first made during the First World War, around 1914 or 1915. "Anzac" stands for Australia and New Zealand Army Corps. Some say they started as cookies made by the troops in the trenches with provisions they had on hand to relieve the boredom of their wartime rations. Others say they were made by resourceful women on the home front who wanted a snack that would keep well during naval transportation to loved ones fighting overseas. The beauty of these cookies is that they are incredibly simple to make—a good recipe for getting your child involved in the kitchen.

¾ cup quick-cooking oats
¾ cup flaked unsweetened coconut
½ cup superfine sugar
¾ cup all-purpose flour
a pinch of salt
7 tablespoons unsalted butter, plus extra for greasing
1 tablespoon golden syrup, such as Lyle's, or light corn syrup
1 teaspoon baking soda
2 tablespoons boiling water

* Preheat the oven to 350°F and grease a couple of baking sheets. Mix the oats, coconut, sugar, flour, and salt in a large bowl. Melt the butter in a small pan and stir in the golden syrup. Add the baking soda to the boiling water and stir this into the golden syrup mixture.
* Make a well in the center of the dry ingredients and pour in the golden syrup mixture. Stir well. Put tablespoons of the dough on the greased baking sheets, placed at least 1 inch apart to allow room for spreading, and flatten the tops slightly.
* Bake for about 10 minutes until golden. Let rest for a few minutes to firm up before transferring to wire racks to cool.

egg-free oat and raisin cookies

There is nothing quite like an egg, especially when it comes to baking. Egg protein is the magical ingredient that holds cookies together and creates light, fluffy sponge cakes. Unfortunately, egg protein is also a potent allergen. Egg substitutes designed mainly for cake making are one solution and can be found at some health-food stores and through specialist suppliers. But they can't mimic the rich flavor that eggs give to cakes, so you may need to add extra butter or flavorings like vanilla. These cookies are quite delicious without egg.

6 tablespoons unsalted butter, softened
½ cup packed light brown sugar
1 tablespoon golden syrup, such as Lyle's, or light corn syrup
1 teaspoon vanilla extract
⅓ cup all-purpose flour
¾ cup quick-cooking oats
¼ teaspoon baking soda
½ teaspoon salt
⅔ cup raisins
⅓ cup pine nuts or sunflower seeds

* Preheat the oven to 350°F.
* Cream the butter, sugar, and golden syrup together until pale and fluffy, then beat in the vanilla. In a separate bowl, stir together the flour, oats, baking soda, and salt, then fold into the butter mixture, followed by the raisins and pine nuts or sunflower seeds.
* Take roughly 2 tablespoons of the mixture and roll into a golf-ball-size ball. Put on lightly greased baking sheets, spaced about 1½ inches apart, and flatten slightly.
* Bake for about 12 minutes, rotating the baking sheets halfway through, until lightly golden. Remove from the oven and allow to cool on the baking sheets for a few minutes, then carefully transfer to cooling racks and allow to cool completely. The cookies will become more crisp as they cool.
* Store in an airtight container for up to 5 days.

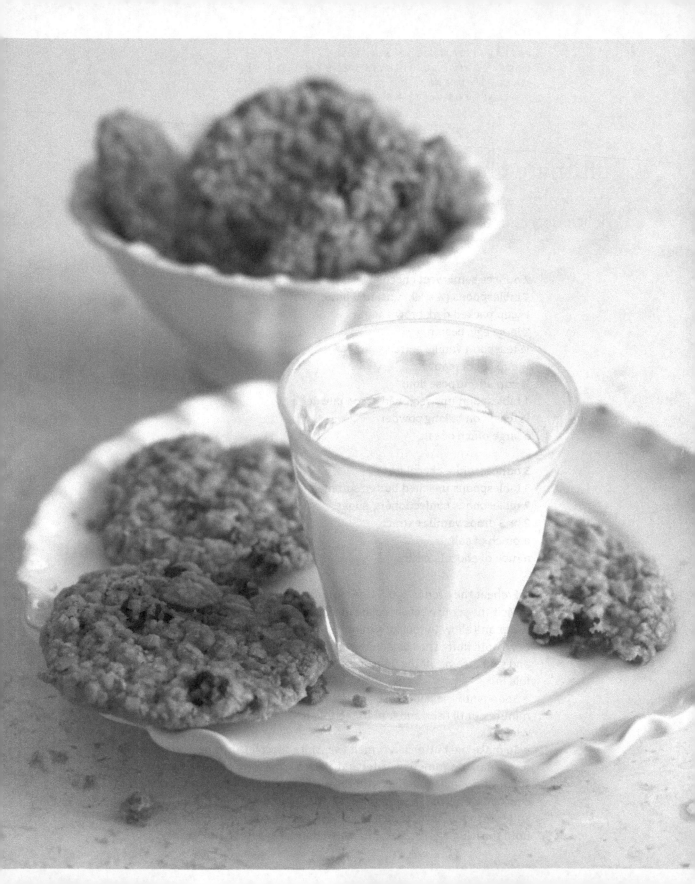

PREPARATION TIME 12 MINUTES
COOKING TIME 20 MINUTES (PLUS CHILLING TIME)
MAKES 8 CUPCAKES
SUITABLE FOR FREEZING (UN-ICED)

ultimate chocolate cupcakes

Fussy eaters are guaranteed to like chocolate, and these are deliciously chocolaty but at the same time light and fluffy.

2 ounces semisweet chocolate

4 tablespoons (½ stick) unsalted butter, softened

⅓ cup packed dark brown sugar

1 large egg, beaten

½ teaspoon vanilla extract

¼ cup sour cream

½ cup all-purpose flour

1 tablespoon unsweetened cocoa powder

½ teaspoon baking powder

a large pinch of salt

WHITE-CHOCOLATE BUTTERCREAM ICING

3 ounces white chocolate

5 tablespoons unsalted butter, softened

2 tablespoons confectioners' sugar

2 or 3 drops vanilla extract

a pinch of salt

a tube of chocolate icing

* Preheat the oven to 350°F. Line a muffin pan with 8 paper cases.
* Melt the semisweet chocolate in a heatproof bowl set over a pan of simmering water and allow to cool for 5 minutes. Cream the butter and brown sugar in a bowl until fluffy, then beat in the cooled chocolate, followed by the egg, vanilla, and sour cream. Sift the flour, cocoa, baking powder, and salt into the bowl and fold in.
* Spoon into the paper cases to around two-thirds full. Bake for 18 to 20 minutes, until risen and firm to the touch. Allow to cool thoroughly on a wire rack.
* To make the buttercream, melt the white chocolate in a heatproof bowl set over a pan of simmering water and allow to cool for 5 minutes. Beat the butter, sugar, and vanilla together with the pinch of salt, then beat in the cooled chocolate. Chill for 20 to 30 minutes, stirring every 10 minutes, until firmer but still spreadable. Swirl the icing over the cupcakes and chill for around 1 hour, until the icing has set. Decorate with chocolate icing, if you like.

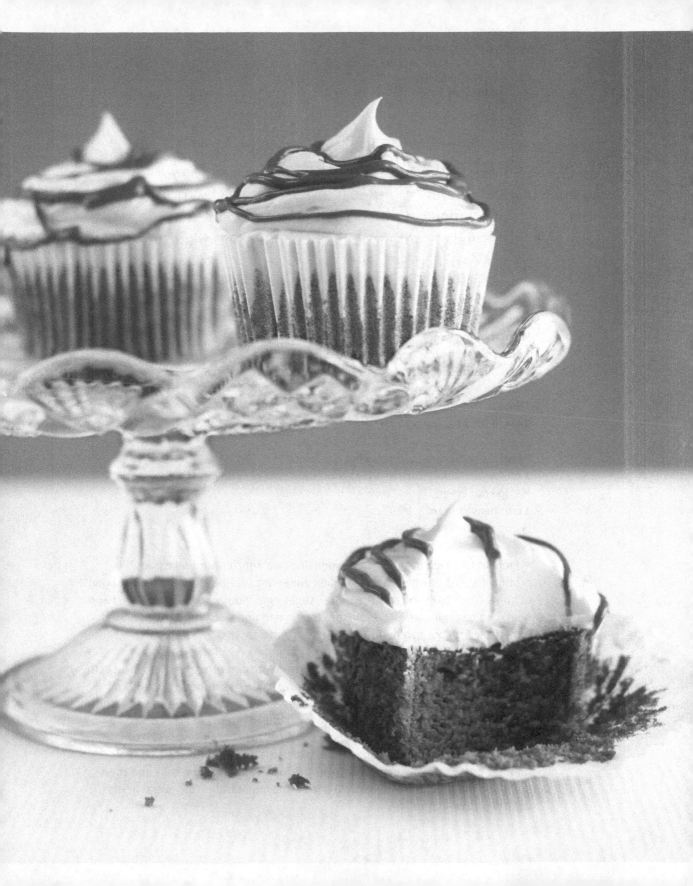

PREPARATION TIME 20 MINUTES
COOKING TIME 20 MINUTES
SERVES 8 TO 10
SUITABLE FOR FREEZING (UN-ICED)

heaven-sent chocolate cake

This cake takes only a few minutes to prepare in an electric mixer, and it is deliciously moist. It's also a fun cake for children to prepare themselves. Chocolate is not all bad, as it contains iron, calcium, and potassium plus a variety of vitamins.

¼ cup unsweetened cocoa powder
¼ cup boiling water
1 stick plus 7 tablespoons unsalted butter, softened
1 cup superfine sugar
4 eggs
1½ cups self-rising flour
2 teaspoons baking powder

CHOCOLATE MOUSSE ICING
7 ounces good-quality semisweet chocolate
2 tablespoons dark rum or 1 teaspoon imitation rum flavoring
½ cup sour cream
1 cup heavy cream
¼ cup crushed M&M's

* Preheat the oven to 350°F. Grease and line two 8-inch round cake pans.
* Stir the cocoa powder into the boiling water until dissolved. Pour into the bowl of an electric mixer and add the butter, sugar, eggs, flour, and baking powder and beat for 2 to 3 minutes. Divide the mixture in half and spoon into the prepared pans. Bake for about 20 minutes, until risen and a toothpick inserted in the center comes out clean. Allow to cool, then turn out onto a wire rack.
* Meanwhile, prepare the icing. Melt the chocolate and rum together with ¼ cup of the sour cream in a heatproof bowl set over a pan of simmering water, and stir until just melted. Remove from the heat, allow to cool a little, and stir in the remaining ¼ cup sour cream. Set aside for about 10 minutes to cool down. Whip the heavy cream until it forms soft peaks, and fold into the chocolate mixture.
* Spread half the icing over one of the cake layers and place the second layer on top. Spread the remaining icing over the top and sides of the cake and then sprinkle the top with crushed M&M's. Set aside in the fridge for several hours until the icing is firm.

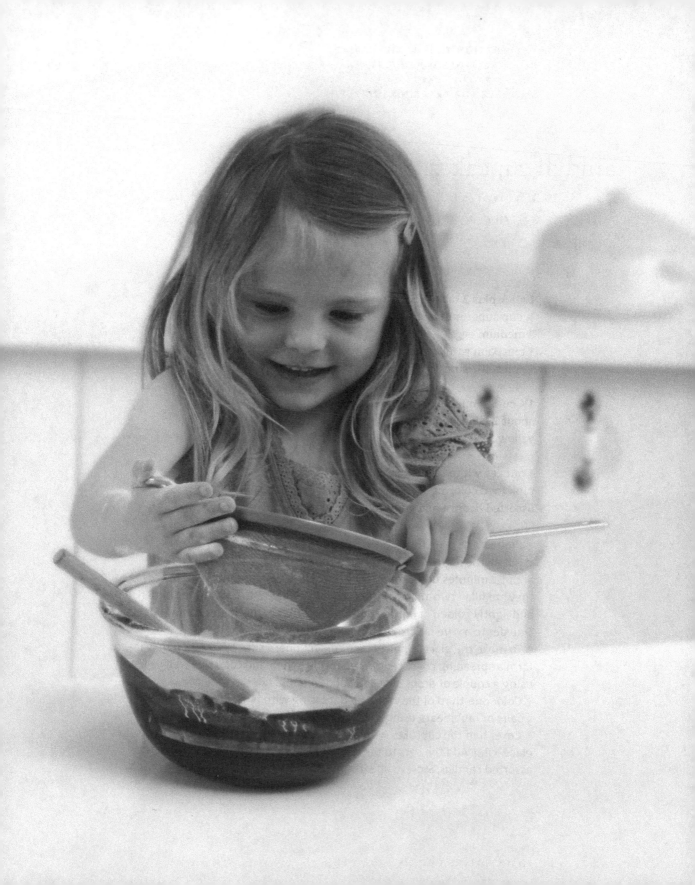

animal cupcakes

Cupcakes are always popular as a snack or for a children's party, and it's fun to decorate them to look like animals, in this case, rabbits and chicks.

1 stick plus 2 tablespoons unsalted butter, softened
¾ cup superfine sugar
3 medium eggs
1 teaspoon vanilla extract
1 cup self-rising flour

GLACÉ ICING
1¼ cups confectioners' sugar, sifted
about 2 tablespoons water
yellow food coloring

DECORATION
4 ounces white rolled fondant icing
pink food coloring
assorted licorice and gumdrop candies

* Preheat the oven to 375°F. Line a muffin pan with 10 paper cases.
* Put all the ingredients for the batter into a mixing bowl and beat for about 2 minutes until smooth. Divide the mixture among the paper cases so they are filled two-thirds of the way up. Bake for 18 to 20 minutes until risen and lightly golden or until a toothpick inserted in the center comes out clean. Transfer to a wire rack to cool.
* To make the glacé icing, mix the confectioners' sugar with enough water to form a spreading consistency, then divide in half and color one-half yellow, using a couple of drops of yellow food coloring.
* Color one-third of the white fondant icing with pink food coloring. Make 5 pairs of rabbit ears, using the white and the pink fondant icing.
* Cover half the cupcakes with the white glacé icing and half with the yellow glacé icing. Add the ears to the white rabbit cupcakes. Decorate with the assorted candies. Store in an airtight container for up to 2 days.

i don't like...

anything homemade

hummingbird cupcakes

Hummingbird cake is a traditional recipe from the American South. No one knows exactly how the name came about, but some say it is because the cake is so good it makes you hum, and so sweet it attracts hummingbirds!

¾ cup all-purpose flour
1 teaspoon baking powder
¼ teaspoon baking soda
1 teaspoon ground ginger
¼ teaspoon salt
¼ cup flaked unsweetened coconut
½ cup packed light brown sugar
1 medium egg, beaten
½ cup canola oil
one 8-ounce can crushed pineapple, drained, 2 tablespoons
    reserved for topping
1 large ripe banana, mashed

TOPPING

4 ounces cream cheese, at room temperature
1 stick unsalted butter, softened
¼ cup confectioners' sugar
3 or 4 drops vanilla extract
2 tablespoons drained canned crushed pineapple, to decorate

* Preheat the oven to 350°F. Line a muffin pan with 8 paper cases.
* Stir together the flour, baking powder, baking soda, ginger, salt, coconut, and sugar. Beat the egg and oil together and add to the dry ingredients, along with the pineapple and banana. Stir together quickly and spoon into the paper cases. Bake for 20 to 25 minutes, until the tops are firm to the touch. Allow to cool on a wire rack.
* To make the topping, beat together the cream cheese, butter, sugar, and vanilla. Spread over the cupcakes and chill until firm. Top with a little of the pineapple just before serving. Store in the fridge.

PREPARATION TIME 25 MINUTES
COOKING TIME 25 MINUTES
MAKES 7 OR 8 PORTIONS
SPONGE SUITABLE FOR FREEZING

sticky toffee pudding cakes

Good old-fashioned comfort food is generally popular as dessert for fussy eaters, and you can't go wrong with this recipe. The sponge and sauce can be made in advance. The sponge also freezes well. Simply thaw, arrange the sponge on a serving plate, pour some sauce on top, and reheat in a microwave (on high), or reheat in the oven, as below, and warm the sauce in a pan.

PUDDING CAKES

4 tablespoons (½ stick) unsalted butter, softened
¾ cup turbinado sugar or granulated sugar
1 tablespoon golden syrup, such as Lyle's, or light corn syrup
1½ tablespoons molasses
2 eggs
1½ cups self-rising flour
1¼ cups boiling water
1 cup pitted dates
1 tablespoon baking soda
½ teaspoon vanilla extract

TOFFEE SAUCE

1 stick unsalted butter
½ cup packed light brown sugar
1 cup heavy cream
a few drops of vanilla extract
a pinch of salt

vanilla ice cream, to serve

* Preheat the oven to 350°F. Spray 7 or 8 small (5-ounce) ramekins or soufflé dishes with nonstick baking spray.
* Cream the butter and sugar together in a food processor. Gradually add the golden syrup, molasses, and eggs. Continue to mix until smooth, then turn down the speed and add the flour, making sure everything is well mixed in.
* Pour the boiling water over the dates and blitz in a blender. Stir in the baking soda and the vanilla. Pour the date puree into the batter while still hot and stir well. Divide the mixture among the ramekins, and bake for 20 to 25 minutes until the tops are just firm to the touch.
* To make the toffee sauce, melt the butter and sugar together in a pan. Add the cream, vanilla, and salt. Bring to a boil, stirring a few times, then simmer for 1 minute.
* Remove the pudding cakes from the ramekins. Place each one on a plate, coat with the warm sauce, and serve with a scoop of vanilla ice cream.

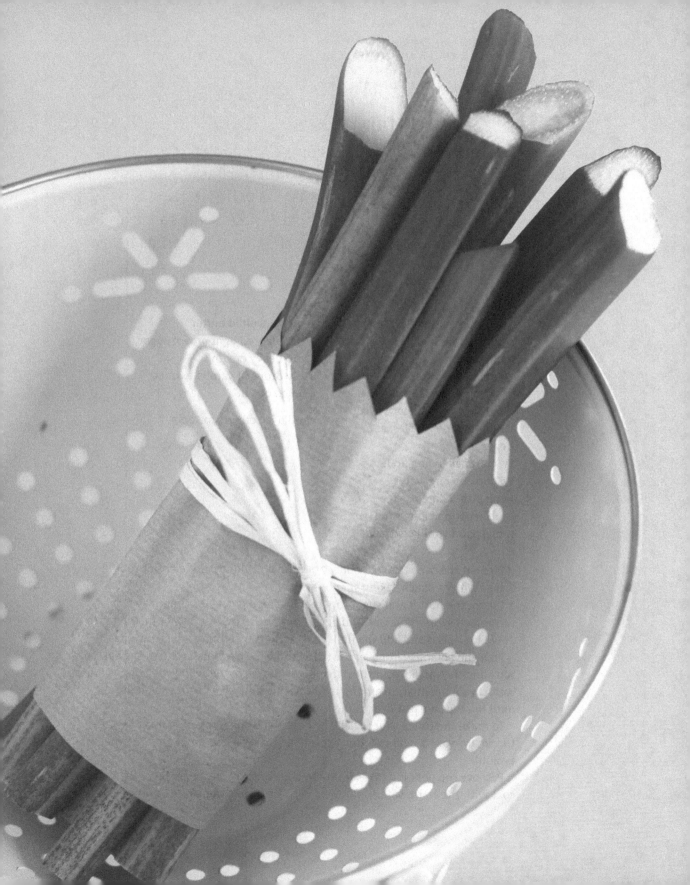

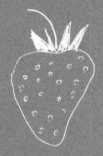

fruity finishes

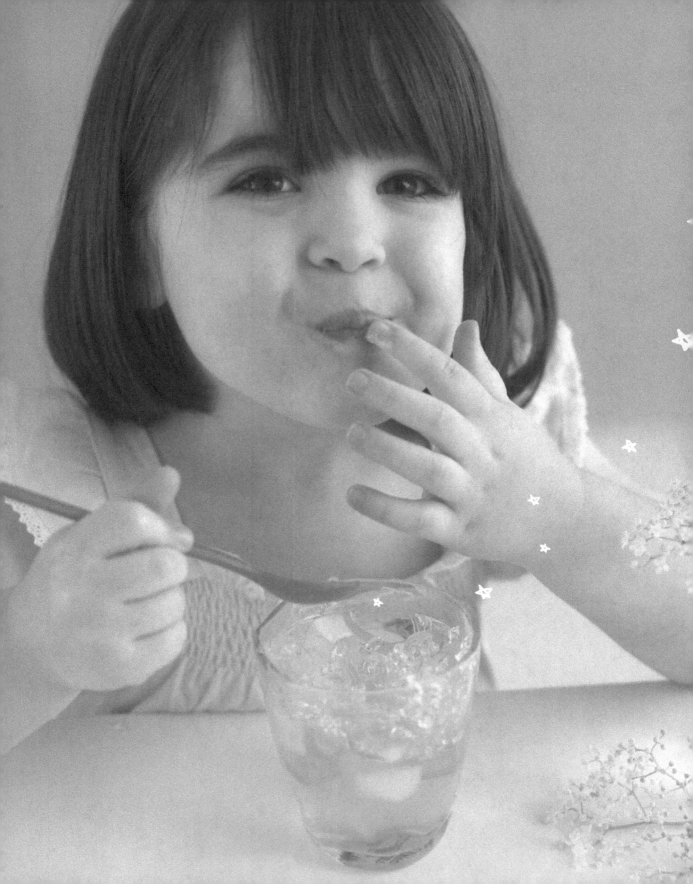

top tips
how to get your child to eat fruit

* Whole fruit in a fruit bowl tends not to get eaten, but how about arranging a plate of colorful cut-up fruit for when your child gets home from school, or even threading some bite-size pieces of fruit onto a straw or a skewer?

* Make sure that any fruit you serve is fully ripe—taste it yourself. Serving unripe, tasteless fruit can put children off.

* Try making fresh-fruit ice pops by blending fresh fruit and mixing with fruit juice or yogurt, then freezing in ice pop molds.

* Find fun ways of serving fruit, like making melon balls; or cut kiwifruit in half and serve in an egg cup. Make a mango hedgehog by cutting the flesh into diagonal cubes and turning inside out.

* Buy a blender and encourage your child to make her own smoothies. In cold weather, serve hot fruity desserts like Rhubarb and Pear Crumble.

* Encourage your child to make her own freshly squeezed orange juice by using an electric citrus juicer.

* Introduce lots of variety—exotic fruits are more readily available in supermarkets, so introduce your child to pitted lychees, passion fruit, mango, or pomegranate.

* Make tasty muffins using fruits like banana and apple and get your child to help make them. Mini muffins are popular, so it's a good idea to buy a mini muffin pan and bake both large and small muffins.

* Add fruit to your child's cereal or make your own delicious granola and add dried fruits.

* Always include some fresh fruit in your child's lunch box. Make sure it is easy to eat—peel fruits such as tangerines and wrap in plastic wrap, and give wedges of melon, mango, etc.

* When you go out, take something fruity with you, such as grapes, a small banana, or dried fruit for when your child is hungry.

Children love gelatin, and combining it with fruit is another good way to up their fruit intake.

PREPARATION TIME 10 MINUTES
  (PLUS CHILLING TIME)
MAKES 4 PORTIONS

PREPARATION TIME 10 MINUTES
COOKING TIME 10 MINUTES
MAKES 2 PORTIONS

gorgeous grape gelatin

You could also use white cranberry juice to make this recipe. If you do, add additional sugar to taste.

3 cups white grape juice
two .25-ounce envelopes unflavored
   gelatin
¼ cup superfine sugar
2 tablespoons fresh lemon juice
1 cup mixed fruit, such as chopped
   peaches (fresh or canned), canned
   fruit cocktail, small halved grapes,
   or a mixture of berries

* Put 1 cup of the grape juice in a pan. Sprinkle the gelatin on top and let stand for 5 minutes. Add the sugar and stir over very low heat until the gelatin has dissolved. Do not allow to boil. Stir in the remaining 2 cups grape juice and the lemon juice. Divide the fruit among four small glasses and pour in the grape juice mixture to fill. Chill for a few hours or overnight, until set.

apples with toffee sauce

This goes well served warm with vanilla ice cream or rice pudding or cold with thick Greek-style yogurt. Alternatively, you could use it as a filling for crepes (see page 28). A combination of warm caramelized fruit with melting cold vanilla ice cream is delectable.

2 medium apples
1 tablespoon unsalted butter
3 tablespoons superfine sugar
¼ cup heavy cream
4 drops of vanilla extract
a pinch of salt

* Peel and core the apples and cut into 12 chunks.
* In a medium pan over medium heat, melt the butter, add the sugar, and cook until the mixture turns to light caramel, 4 to 5 minutes.
* Stir in the cream and apples, and simmer for 3 to 4 minutes until the apples are tender. Remove from the heat and stir in the vanilla and salt.

tropical fruit salad

Sadly, whole fruit in a fruit bowl rarely gets eaten. This lovely fruit salad is a good way to tempt fussy eaters.

¼ cup tropical fruit juice
¼ cup sugar
2 teaspoons fresh lime juice
1 medium mango, peeled, flesh cut into cubes
½ small pineapple, peeled, cored, and cubed
1 papaya, seeded, peeled, and diced

* Put the juice in a small pan with the sugar and 2 tablespoons water and stir over low heat until the sugar has dissolved. Bring to a boil and cook for 30 seconds. Allow to cool and add the lime juice.
* Put the fruit in a large bowl and pour the syrup over it. Allow to stand for 30 minutes before serving.

☆ Try to give your child a wide variety of fruits, as different fruits provide different nutrients. For example, a single kiwifruit supplies more than the normal daily requirement of vitamin C for an adult, while mango is a very rich source of beta-carotene (vitamin A), which is essential for growth, healthy skin, fighting infection, and good vision. It may seem obvious, but if you want your child to enjoy eating fruit, do make sure the fruit is ripe. Other fruits you could add are pitted lychees or cantaloupe, which looks good if you scoop out the flesh using a melon baller.

apple and blackberry crisp

Crisps are surprisingly easy to make, as you can whiz up the topping in a food processor—take care not to overmix. Alternatively, children might have more fun helping you make the topping by hand.

3 tablespoons unsalted butter
2 pounds eating apples (such as Gala, Pink Lady, and Fuji), peeled, cored, and sliced about ¼ inch thick
2½ tablespoons light brown sugar
12 ounces fresh or frozen blackberries

TOPPING
1¾ cups all-purpose flour
a good pinch of salt
1 teaspoon ground cinnamon
1 stick unsalted cold butter, cubed
½ cup superfine sugar
3 tablespoons light brown sugar

* You will need an 8-inch square ovenproof dish.
* Preheat the oven to 400°F.
* Melt the butter in a large pan and sauté the apples for 1 minute. Sprinkle with the sugar and continue to cook for 2 minutes more. Stir in the blackberries. Spoon the fruit into the ovenproof dish.
* To make the topping, mix together the flour, salt, and ½ teaspoon of the cinnamon. Rub in the butter, then stir in the superfine sugar. Alternatively, whiz together in a food processor for a few seconds.
* Sprinkle the topping over the fruit. Mix the remaining ½ teaspoon cinnamon with the brown sugar and sprinkle over the crisp. Bake for 40 minutes.

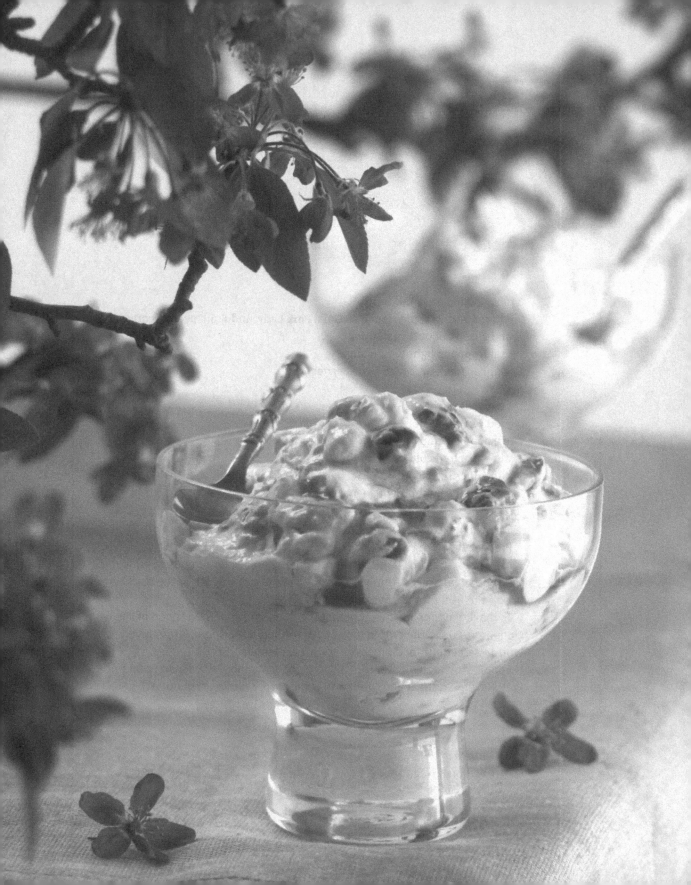

annabel's berry mess

Meringue tends to be popular with children, so try combining it with berries—the combination of slightly tart berries with crushed meringue is heavenly. Berries are very rich in vitamin C, which helps us to fight infection and absorb iron. You could also puree and strain some raspberries, mix together with a little confectioners' sugar to make a raspberry coulis, and stir this through the mixture. Raspberry coulis is another way to boost your child's vitamin-C levels, and it goes well with vanilla ice cream and peaches to make a peach Melba.

8 ounces mixed berries (such as blueberries, blackberries,
    strawberries, and raspberries)
1 tablespoon plus 1 teaspoon confectioners' sugar
½ cup heavy cream
¼ teaspoon vanilla extract
one 6-ounce container Greek-style yogurt
6 meringue kiss cookies, broken into small pieces

* Put the berries in a bowl. Add the 1 tablespoon sugar and mix, crushing a few of the berries. In a separate bowl, combine the cream, the 1 teaspoon sugar, and the vanilla, and whip to soft peaks.
* Stir the yogurt to loosen slightly, then carefully fold into the cream, followed by the berries and the meringue pieces. Spoon the mixture into 4 glasses and serve.
* You can chill this for up to 30 minutes but not much longer, otherwise the meringue will start to get soggy.

annabel's berry ~~mess~~ mess

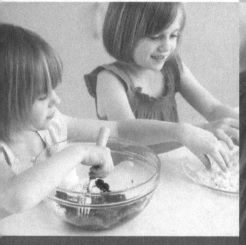

TIP
When children cook, they learn skills like counting, measuring, weighing, and understanding time—all without noticing.

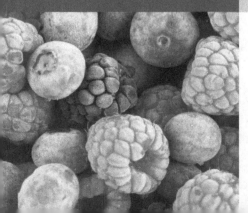

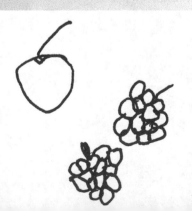

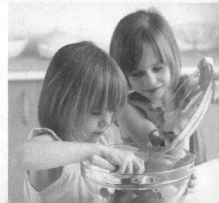

PREPARATION TIME 15 MINUTES
COOKING TIME 50 MINUTES
MAKES 6 PORTIONS

mini meringue pavlova

Pavlova is a meringue dessert named after ballet dancer
Anna Pavlova. The meringue is crisp on the outside but chewy
on the inside. It's very popular with children and fun for them
to make themselves.

MERINGUE
2 large egg whites
½ teaspoon cornstarch
½ teaspoon fresh lemon juice
a pinch of salt
½ cup superfine sugar

TOPPING
¾ cup raspberries, plus extra for decoration
1½ tablespoons confectioners' sugar
⅓ cup mascarpone cheese
mint leaves for decoration (optional)

* Preheat the oven to 230°F.
* Cut a piece of baking parchment to fit a large baking sheet. Draw six 4-inch-diameter circles on the paper (use a large cup or ramekin as a template) and put the parchment on the baking sheet, pen side down, so you don't get ink on the meringue. Alternatively, use an ice-cream scoop to form the meringues.
* Whisk the egg whites with the cornstarch, lemon juice, and salt until the mixture forms stiff peaks. Add one-third of the sugar and whisk until it reaches stiff peaks again. Repeat with another third of the sugar, then whisk in the final third of sugar.
* Spoon the meringue into the centers of the circles and spread out, using the circles as a guide. Make a little indentation in the center of each using the back of a teaspoon. Bake for about 50 minutes until crisp on the outside and dry underneath. Allow to cool, then gently peel off the paper.
* Mash the raspberries with the confectioners' sugar. Stir half into the mascarpone, then ripple through the remaining raspberries. Spoon a little of the mixture into the middle of the meringues, and decorate with the extra raspberries and maybe a couple of mint leaves if you like.

rhubarb and pear crumble

If your child isn't keen on eating fruit, you might be able to tempt him or her with this fruity crumble—it's one of my favorites. Rhubarb is great for making crumbles, as the slightly tart fruit combines well with the sweet crumble topping. And, hey, a little secret—strictly speaking, rhubarb is a vegetable, so you have managed to get your child to eat fruit *and* a vegetable. I put almond flour into the dish before I add the fruit, as this helps to soak up some of the juices and stop the crumble from becoming soggy.

2 tablespoons unsalted butter
½ teaspoon ground ginger
¼ cup turbinado sugar or granulated sugar
4 ripe pears, peeled, cored, and cut into chunks
¾ pound rhubarb, cut into ½-inch pieces
2 tablespoons almond flour

CRUMBLE TOPPING
½ cup quick-cooking oats
¾ cup all-purpose flour
⅓ cup crumbled amaretti cookies
a large pinch of salt
6 tablespoons cold unsalted butter, cut into cubes
¼ cup turbinado sugar or granulated sugar

* Preheat the oven to 400°F. Melt the butter in a large pan, add the ginger and sugar, and allow to dissolve. Add the pears and cook on low heat for 2 minutes or until softened. Stir in the rhubarb and cook for 2 minutes. Sprinkle the bottom of an 8-inch square ovenproof dish (or 6 individual dishes) with the almond flour and spoon the fruit on top.
* To make the topping, put the oats, flour, amaretti cookies, and salt in the bowl of a food processor and whiz into crumbs. Add the butter and pulse until it has disappeared, then add the sugar and pulse once or twice to combine.
* Spread the topping over the fruit and bake in the center of the oven for about 35 minutes until lightly golden.

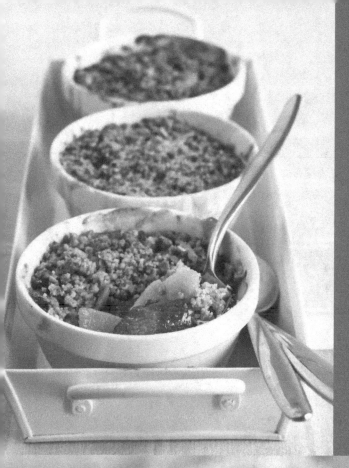

i don't like...

any
hot fruit

:(

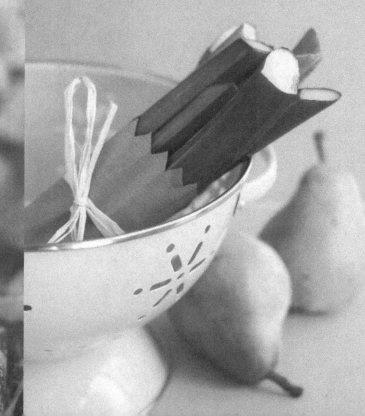

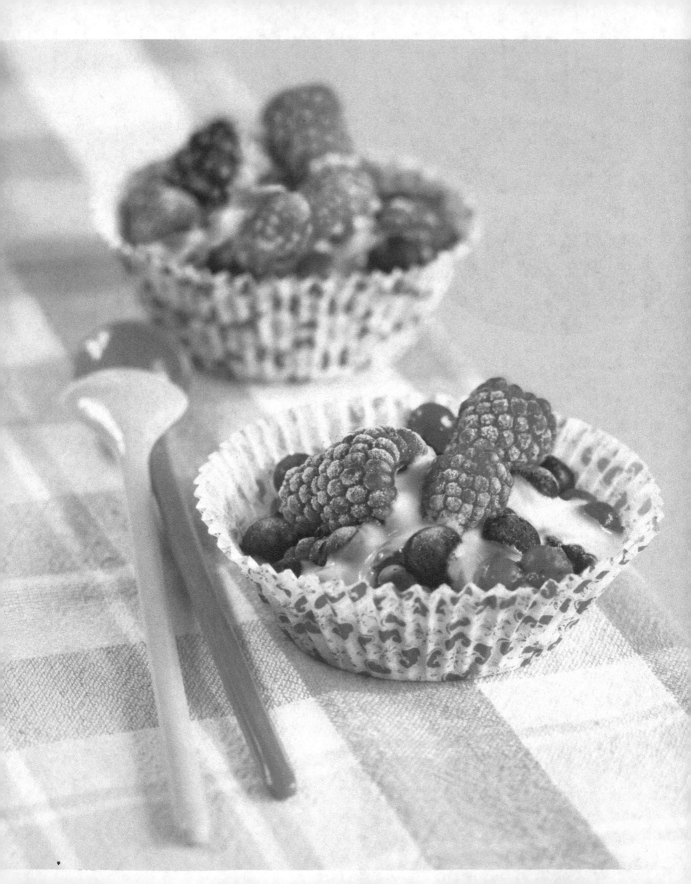

frozen berries with hot white-chocolate sauce

This is served up in some of the poshest restaurants as dessert, but it's dead simple to make at home and oh so plate-lickingly good that I defy the fussiest eater to refuse it! It's best to freeze the berries yourself, as ready-frozen berries tend to get a bit mushy when thawed. This is a particular favorite of my daughter Lara, who has always been a bit fussy. She was the inspiration behind the "I don't like . . ." lists in this book.

1¼ cups mixed berries (such as blackberries, raspberries, blueberries, strawberries, and red currants)
2 ounces white chocolate, chopped into small pieces
¼ cup heavy cream

* To freeze the berries, line a rimmed baking sheet with baking parchment or waxed paper and arrange the berries in a single layer. When they are frozen, transfer to small freezer bags. They will last for 1 month and are also good in smoothies.
* Take the berries out of the freezer and divide between two bowls. Allow them to thaw slightly at room temperature for about 10 minutes.
* Put the chocolate and cream in a microwavable bowl and cook for 10 seconds, stir, and repeat heating and stirring until the chocolate has just melted (it will take 4 or 5 blasts) and you have a smooth sauce. Alternatively, put the chocolate and cream in a small heatproof bowl over a pan of simmering water and stir continuously until the chocolate has just melted.
* Pour the hot sauce immediately over the berries and serve at once.

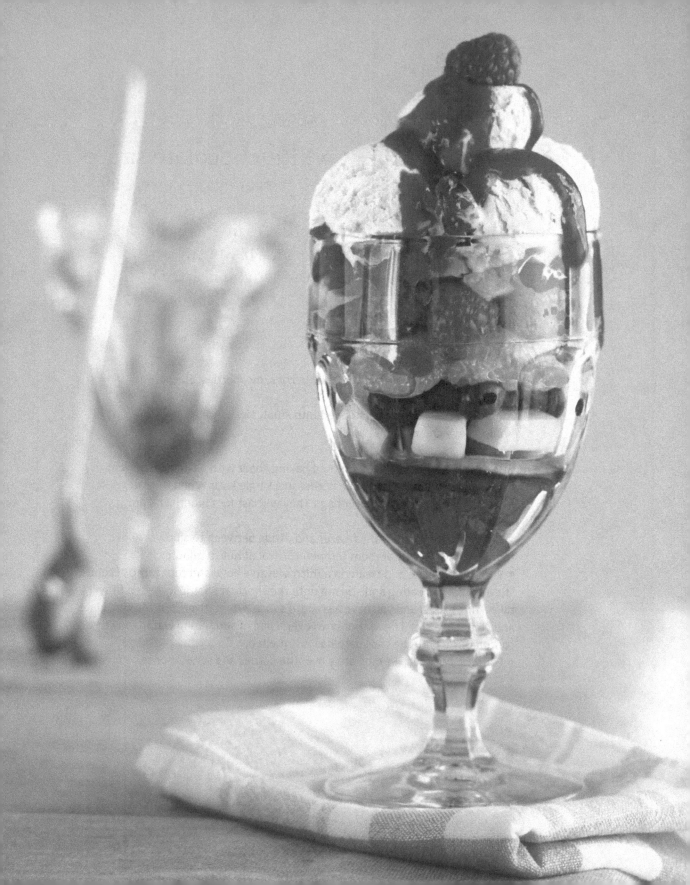

knickerbocker glory parfait

Let your child make up her own combination of gelatin, fruit, and ice cream. Old-fashioned long stockings with colorful stripes were called knickerbockers, and that's how this parfait got its name.

1 pint good-quality vanilla ice cream

GELATIN

one 3-ounce package cranberry Jell-O
1 cup cold 7UP

RASPBERRY SAUCE

1 cup raspberries
2 tablespoons confectioners' sugar
½ teaspoon fresh lemon juice

PLUS TWO OR THREE OF THE FOLLOWING:

3 ripe kiwifruits, peeled and diced
1½ cups mixed berries
3 rings fresh or canned pineapple, diced
½ large ripe mango, peeled, flesh diced
one 11-ounce can mandarin oranges, drained

* Prepare the Jell-O according to the package directions, but use the 7UP in place of the second cup of water. Pour into a bowl, pop in the fridge, and chill for 4 to 5 hours or overnight, until set. When set, you can chop some of the gelatin into pieces.
* To make the sauce, blend the raspberries, sugar, and lemon juice. Strain to remove seeds and chill until needed.
* To construct the Knickerbocker Glories, divide the gelatin among 4 sundae glasses. Layer the fruit over the gelatin. Add another layer of chopped gelatin and top with scoops of ice cream. Finally, pour the raspberry puree on top. Serve with long spoons.

ice pops

What child can resist an ice pop? It's so easy to make your own from good healthy ingredients like pureed fruits, fruit juice, or yogurt. You could simply freeze your child's favorite juice or fruit smoothie in ice pop molds. If you have time, you could freeze in two stages using contrasting colors to make a two-tone ice pop. Pour in the strawberry mix up to halfway, then freeze for a couple of hours and fill to the top with the tropical mix, or use tropical fruit juice. Add the sticks, and when they're frozen, you'll have red and orange pops.

strawberry sorbet ice pops

Strawberries contain higher levels of vitamin C than any other berries.

2 tablespoons superfine sugar
8 ounces strawberries, halved
juice of 1 medium orange (about ¼ cup)

* Put the sugar and ¼ cup water in a saucepan and boil until syrupy (about 3 minutes). Allow to cool.
* Puree the strawberries with a handheld electric blender and combine with the cooled syrup and orange juice, then pour this mixture into 4 large ice pop molds. Freeze until solid.

tropical pops

1 large mango, peeled and diced
¾ cup tropical fruit juice
3 tablespoons confectioners' sugar
1 tablespoon fresh lemon juice

* Blend the ingredients together until smooth. Pour into 4 large ice pop molds and freeze.

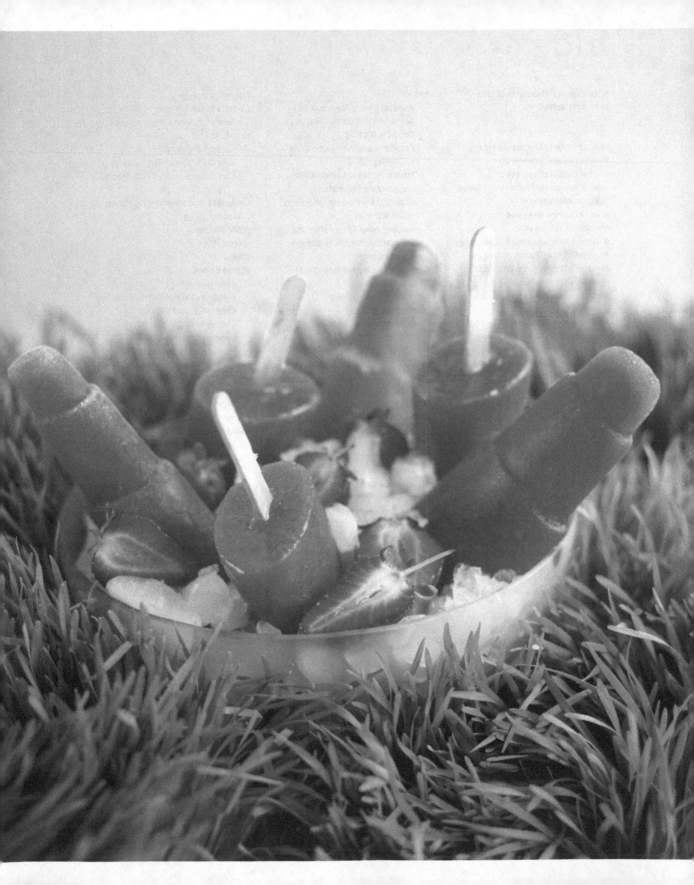

index

Note: Page numbers in **bold** refer to photographs.

additives 11
Alison's Favorite Shepherd's Pie 139
Almost Instant Oatmeal 20
Animal Cupcakes 194, **195**
Animal Pasta Salad with Multicolored Vegetables **102**, 103
Annabel's Berry Mess **206**, 207
Annabel's Granola **18**, 19
Annabel's Mini Vegetable Burgers 40, **41**
Annabel's Secret Tomato Sauce 45
Annabel's Tasty Shrimp Wrap 67
Annabel's Yummy Burgers 138
Anzac Cookies **186**, 187
apples
    Apple and Blackberry Crisp 205
    Apples with Toffee Sauce 203
    French Toast with Caramelized Apples 26, **27**
    Oat, Apple, and Sunflower Seed Muffins 183
    Pork Medallions with Caramelized Apples 148
apricot buttercream 182
Arugula and Cherry Tomatoes, Chicken Paillard with **126**, 127
attention spans 15

babies, weaning 9
Bacon and Tomato Spaghetti Sauce 104
Bag-Baked Cod Niçoise 84, **85**
balsamic vinegar 58
bananas
    Bananarama 25
    Jamaican Banana Muffins **180**, 181
    smoothies 23, 25
    toffee-banana topping 29
Barbecue Dip 125
Barbecue Sauce 133, 146
barbecues 10
batter 36
béchamel sauce 96
beef
    Alison's Favorite Shepherd's Pie 139
    Annabel's Yummy Burgers 138
    Hidden Vegetable Spaghetti Bolognese 91
    Meatballs with Tomato Sauce 136, **137**
    Mini Meat Loaves 144
    Nicholas's Lasagne 96
    Sloppy Joe 149
    Swedish Meatballs 145
    Teriyaki Beef Skewers 142, **143**

berries
    Annabel's Berry Mess **206**, 207
    Apple and Blackberry Crisp 205
    Berry Burst **22**, 23
    Cranberry and White Chocolate Cookies 168
    Frozen Berries with Hot White-Chocolate Sauce **212**, 213
    Grace's Dairy-Free Summer Berry Smoothie 25
    Knickerbocker Glory Parfait **214**, 215
    see also blueberries; raspberries; strawberries
Birthday Cake, Wheat-Free 170–71
birthday parties 7
blind man's grub game 9
blueberries
    blueberry compote 26
    Blueberry Muffins 169
Bolognese, Hidden Vegetable Spaghetti 91
bran
    Raisin Bran Breakfast Muffins 30, **31**
breakfast
    fruit for 201
    general recipes 13–33
    gluten-free recipes 155
    on the run 15, 32
    wraps 32, **33**
Brownies, Gluten-Free 166, **167**
burgers 9
    Annabel's Mini Vegetable Burgers 40, **41**
    Annabel's Yummy Burgers 138
    Yummy Vegetable and Cashew Nut Burgers 38, **39**
buttercream
    apricot 182
    chocolate 170–71
    vanilla 170–71
    white-chocolate 190, **191**
Butternut Squash Risotto 37

Caesar Dressing, Creamy 57
cakes 154
    Animal Cupcakes 194, **195**
    Carrot Bar Cake 177
    gluten-free **164**, 165, 166, **167**
    Gluten-Free Brownies 166, **167**
    Heaven-sent Chocolate Cake 192, **193**
    Hummingbird Cupcakes 196
    Perfect Lemon Polenta Cake **164**, 165
    Ultimate Chocolate Cupcakes 190, **191**
    Vanilla Cupcakes 171
    Wheat-Free Birthday Cake 170–71
    Yogurt "Pot" Cupcakes 182
    see also muffins

Cannelloni 52–53
carbohydrates, complex 15, 17
Caroline's Lasagne Alfredo 106, **107**
carrots 36
    Carrot Bar Cake 177
    Carrot and Cucumber Salad 55
    Carrot Spice Cookies with Maple Fudge Glaze 176
Cashew Nut and Yummy Vegetable Burgers 38, **39**
celiac disease 153–54
cereals 15
challah 26
cheese dishes
    Cannelloni 52–53
    Caroline's Lasagne Alfredo 106, **107**
    Cheesy Choux Puffs 160
    Cheesy Mini Quiches **156**, 157
    Cheesy Zucchini Sticks 46
    Focaccia Pizza 42–44, **43–44**
    Kiddie Carbonara 105
    Mighty Mac and Cheese **100**, 101
    Polenta Mini Pizzas 162, **163**
    Vegetable Quesadillas 50, **51**
cheese sauce 100, 106
chicken 109–33
    Animal Pasta Salad with Multicolored Vegetables **102**, 103
    Caroline's Lasagne Alfredo 106, **107**
    Chicken Balls in Tomato Sauce 132
    Chicken Drumsticks with Barbecue Sauce 133
    Chicken and Leek Pie with Potato Pastry 158–59
    Chicken Nuggets with Dipping Sauces **124**, 125
    Chicken Paillard with Arugula and Cherry Tomatoes **126**, 127
    Chicken Satay Skewers 123
    Chicken in Tomato and Sweet Pepper Sauce 131
    Chinese Chicken Wraps 112, **113**
    Hawaiian Chicken Salad 54
    Japanese Chicken Salad **116**, 117
    Japanese-Style Chicken Fillets 111
    Lara's Chicken Wraps 114–15
    Maple-Glazed Grilled Chicken 120, **121**
    Marina's Pasta with Pesto and Cherry Tomatoes 97
    Mini Chicken Patties 110
    Monday-Night Risotto 119
    Mummy's Ramen Noodles 92, **93**
    Nasi Goreng: Indonesian Fried Rice 118
    One-Bowl Meal 133
    Sticky Chicken 122
    Ten-Minute Chicken Noodle Soup 115

Yummy Chicken Quesadillas 128, **129–30**
chicken nuggets 9, **124**, 125
Chinese Chicken Wraps 112, **113**
Chinese-Style Sauce 87
chips
    Root Vegetable Oven Fries 61
    Vegetable Chips 60
Chive Sauce 74
chocolate
    chocolate buttercream 170–71
    chocolate mousse icing 192
    Chocolate Pudding Cakes with Chocolate Fudge Sauce 184–85, **184–85**
    Cranberry and White Chocolate Cookies 168
    Flourless Peanut Butter and Chocolate Chip Cookies 161
    Frozen Berries with Hot White-Chocolate Sauce **212**, 213
    Gluten-Free Brownies 166, **167**
    Heaven-sent Chocolate Cake 192, **193**
    Ultimate Chocolate Cupcakes 190, **191**
choice 11
chutney, Mrs Ball's 122
cod
    Bag-Baked Cod Niçoise 84, **85**
    Crunchy Popcorn Fish **82**, 83
    Drunken Fish with Little Trees 87
    Fabulous Fish Pie 75
    Golden Fish Sticks **80**, 81
    Mini Fish Pies 76–77, **77**
    Salmon and Cod in a Chive Sauce 74
    Sweet-and-sour Fish 86
concentration 15
Confetti Couscous Salad **48**, 49
cookies
    Anzac Cookies **186**, 187
    Carrot Spice Cookies with Maple Fudge Glaze 176
    Cranberry and White Chocolate Cookies 168
    Egg-Free Oat and Raisin Cookies 188, **189**
    Flourless Peanut Butter and Chocolate Chip Cookies 161
    My Favorite Gingersnaps **178**, 179
    Trail Mix Bars 174, **175**
cooking with children 7
Corn Fritters, Mini 62, **63**
Couscous Salad, Confetti **48**, 49
Cranberry and White Chocolate Cookies 168
Creamy Caesar Dressing 57
crepes

My Favorite 28–29
toppings 29
Crisp, Apple and Blackbery, 205
crudités 36
Crumble, Rhubarb and Pear 210, **211**
Crunchy Popcorn Fish **82**, 83
Cucumber and Carrot Salad 55
cupcakes
    Animal 194, **195**
    Vanilla 171
    Yogurt "Pot" 182

dairy-free foods 25, 155
dentists 10
desserts
    cookies and cakes 173–97
    fruit recipes 199–219
    gluten-free 161, **164**, 165–71, **167**
dips
    barbecue 125
    herby ranch 58
    honey-mustard 125
drinks 10
    see also smoothies
Drunken Fish with Little Trees 87

Eat Up books 8
edamame beans 111
Egg-Free Oat and Raisin Cookies 188, **189**
eggs
    for breakfast 15
    Cheesy Mini Quiches **156**, 157
    Frittata 47
    nutritional value of 21
    Omelet Crepe 21
Enchiladas, Yummy Chicken 128, **129–30**

Fabulous Fish Pie 75
family mealtimes 7
fish recipes 65–87
Fish Sticks, Golden **80**, 81
fish cakes
    Salmon Fish Cakes 73
    Tuna Melt Fish Cakes 72
flexible eating 15
Flourless Peanut Butter and Chocolate Chip Cookies 161
flours, gluten-free 154
Focaccia Pizza 42–44, **43–44**
food intolerances 153–54
French Toast with Caramelized Apples 26, **27**
Fresh Tomato Sauce for Spaghetti 98
Frittata 47
Fritters, Mini Corn 62, **63**
Frozen Berries with Hot White-Chocolate Sauce **212**, 213

fruit
    dippers 32
    Fruity Muesli **16**, 17
    getting children to eat 201
    ice pops 201, 216, **217**
    muffins 32, 201
    recipes 199–219
    wraps 32

games 10
    blind man's grub 9
    food detective 11
gelatin
    Georgeous Grape Gelatin **202**, 203
    Knickerbocker Glory Parfait **214**, 215
Gingersnaps, My Favorite **178**, 179
Gluten-Free Brownies 166, **167**
gluten-free recipes 4, 151–71, 181
Golden Fish Sticks **80**, 81
Grace's Dairy-Free Summer Berry Smoothie 25
Grace's Dairy- and Gluten-Free Bircher Muesli 155
granola 32
    Annabel's Granola **18**, 19
Gray, Rose 165
guacamole 50

ham
    Kiddie Carbonara 105
    Hawaiian Chicken Salad 54
    Heaven-sent Chocolate Cake 192, **193**
    Herby Ranch Dressing 58
    Hidden Vegetable Spaghetti Bolognese 91
    honey-mustard dip 125
    Hummingbird Cupcakes 196

ice cream
    Knickerbocker Glory Parfait **214**, 215
ice pops 201
    Strawberry Sorbet 216, **217**
    Tropical Pops 216
icing 177, 196
    chocolate mousse icing 192
    cream cheese icing 177
    glacé icing 194, **195**
    see also buttercream
Indonesian Fried Rice: Nasi Goreng 118
iron 15, 19, 21

Jamaican Banana Muffins 180, 181
Japanese Chicken Salad **116**, 117
Japanese-Style Chicken Fillets 111
junk foods, healthy versions 4, 9
    Chicken Nuggets with Dipping Sauces **124**, 125
    Mummy's Ramen Noodles 92, **93**
    see also burgers; pizzas

Kebabs, Vegetable 54
Kiddie Carbonara 105
Knickerbocker Glory Parfait **214**, 215

lamb
   Alison's Favorite Shepherd's Pie 139
   Lamb Lollipops 149
   Luscious Lamb Koftas **140**, 141
Lara's Chicken Wraps 114–15
Lasagne, Nicholas's 96
Lasagne Alfredo, Caroline's 106, **107**
lecithin 21
Leek and Chicken Pie with Potato Pastry
   158–59
Lemon Polenta Cake, Perfect **164**, 165
lunch boxes 10, 201
Luscious Lamb Koftas **140**, 141

macaroni and cheese **100**, 101
malnutrition 4
Maple Fudge Glaze, Carrot Spice Cookies
   with 176
Maple-Glazed Grilled Chicken 120, **121**
marinades
   for Chicken Drumsticks 133
   for Chicken Nuggets 125
   for Chicken Paillard with Arugula
      and Cherry Tomatoes 127
   for Chicken Satay Skewers 123
   for Lara's Chicken Wraps 114–15
   for Maple-Glazed Grilled Chicken 120
   for Sticky Chicken 122
Marina's Pasta with Pesto and Cherry
   Tomatoes 97
Mascarpone and Tomato Sauce, Pasta
   with **94**, 95
meal-skipping 15
meals on the run 15, 32
meat recipes 135–49
Meatballs with Tomato Sauce 136, **137**
meringues
   Annabel's Berry Mess **206**, 207
   Mini Meringue Pavlova **208**, 209
Mighty Mac and Cheese **100**, 101
Mini Chicken Patties 110
Mini Corn Fritters 62, **63**
Mini Fish Pies 76–77, **77**
Mini Meat Loaves 144
Mini Meringue Pavlova **208**, 209
Monday-Night Risotto 119
Mrs Ball's chutney 122
muesli
   Fruity Muesli **16**, 17
   Grace's Dairy- and Gluten-Free
      Bircher Muesli 155
muffins
   Blueberry Muffins 169
   fruit 32, 201

Jamaican Banana Muffins **180**, 181
Oat, Apple, and Sunflower Seed
   Muffins 183
Raisin Bran Breakfast Muffins 30,
   31
Mummy's Ramen Noodles 92, **93**
My Favorite Gingersnaps **178**, 179
My Favorite Crepes 28–29

Nasi Goreng: Indonesian Fried Rice 118
neophobia 11
Nicholas's Lasagne 96
no, learning to say 11
noodles
   Mummy's Ramen Noodles 92,
      93
   Pork and Peanut Noodles 90
   Salmon on a Stick with Stir-fried
      Noodles 70, **71**
   Ten-Minute Chicken Noodle Soup
      115

Oatmeal, Almost Instant 20
oats
   Annabel's Granola **18**, 19
   Egg-Free Oat and Raisin Cookies 188,
      189
   Oat, Apple, and Sunflower Seed
      Muffins 183
obese children 4
One-Bowl Meal 133
orange
   Sunshine Smoothie 23
Oriental Salad 69
Orzo Salad 55
overweight children 4

packed lunches 10, 201
paprika, smoked 120
pasta dishes 52–53, 55, 89–107
Pasta with Tomato and Mascarpone
   Sauce **94**, 95
pastry 154
   Cheesy Mini Quiches **156**, 157
   Chicken and Leek Pie with Potato
      Pastry 158–59
Pavlova, Mini Meringue **208**, 209
Peanut Butter and Chocolate Chip
   Cookies, Flourless 161
Peanut and Pork Noodles 90
pears
   Rhubarb and Pear Crumble 210,
      211
Perfect Lemon Polenta Cake **164**, 165
Pesto and Cherry Tomatoes, Marina's
   Pasta with 97
picnics 10

pies
   Alison's Favorite Shepherd's Pie 139
   Chicken and Leek Pie with Potato
      Pastry 158–59
   Fabulous Fish Pie 75
   fish 66, 75, 76–77, **77**
   Mini Fish Pies 76–77, **77**
pine nuts 49
pineapple
   Sunshine Smoothie 23
pizzas 9
   Focaccia Pizza 42–44, **43–44**
   Polenta Mini Pizzas 162, **163**
polenta
   Perfect Lemon Polenta Cake **164**, 165
   Polenta Mini Pizzas 162, **163**
pork
   Pork Medallions with Caramelized
      Apples 148
   Pork and Peanut Noodles 90
   Sticky BBQ Ribs 146, **147**
   Swedish Meatballs 145
portion sizes 8, 9
potatoes
   Alison's Favorite Shepherd's Pie 139
   Annabel's Mini Vegetable Burgers 40
   Chicken and Leek Pie with Potato
      Pastry 158–59
   Fabulous Fish Pie 75
   Frittata 47
   mashed 36
   Mini Fish Pies 76–77, **77**
   Spicy Potato Wedges 61
presentation of food 9
processed foods 154
protein 15, 21

Quesadillas
   Vegetable 50, **51**
Quiches, Cheesy Mini **156**, 157

raisins
   Egg-Free Oat and Raisin Cookies 188,
      189
   Raisin Bran Breakfast Muffins 30, **31**
raspberries
   Knickerbocker Glory Parfait **214**, 215
   Mini Meringue Pavlova **208**, 209
raw foods 36
reward schemes 8
Rhubarb and Pear Crumble 210, **211**
rice dishes
   Butternut Squash Risotto 37
   Japanese Chicken Salad **116**, 117
   Monday-Night Risotto 119
   Nasi Goreng: Indonesian Fried Rice
      118

Rogers, Ruth 165
Root Vegetable Oven Fries 61

salad dressings 36, 57–58, 103, 117, 127
salads 36
    Animal Pasta Salad with
        Multicolored Vegetables **102**, 103
    Carrot and Cucumber Salad 55
    Confetti Couscous Salad **48**, 49
    Hawaiian Chicken Salad 54
    Japanese Chicken Salad **116**, 117
    Oriental Salad 59
    Orzo Salad 55
salmon
    Crunchy Popcorn Fish **82**, 83
    Fabulous Fish Pie 75
    Mini Fish Pies 76–77, **77**
    Salmon and Cod in a Chive Sauce 74
    Salmon Fish Cakes 73
    Salmon on a Stick with Stir-fried
        Noodles 70, **71**
    Super Salmon Wrap 67
sardines 66
Satay Skewers, Chicken 123
sauces
    Annabel's Secret Tomato Sauce 45
    Bacon and Tomato Spaghetti Sauce
        104
    Barbecue Sauce 133, 146
    béchamel sauce 96
    cheese sauce 100, 106
    Chinese-Style Sauce 87
    Chive Sauce 74
    Chocolate Fudge Sauce 184–85,
        184–85
    Fresh Tomato Sauce for Spaghetti 98
    Hot White-Chocolate Sauce **212**, 213
    for Japanese-Style Chicken Fillets 111
    Kiddie Carbonara 105
    for Mini Fish Pies 76–77, **77**
    raspberry sauce **214**, 215
    for Swedish Meatballs 145
    Sweet-and-sour Sauce 86
    tartar sauce 81
    Teriyaki Sauce 142, **143**
    Toffee Sauce 197, 203
    Tomato and Mascarpone Sauce **94**,
        95
    Tomato Sauce 132, 136
    Tomato and Sweet Pepper Sauce 131
    white sauce 75
shrimp
    Annabel's Tasty Shrimp Wrap 67
    Nasi Goreng: Indonesian Fried Rice 118
    Shrimp Toasts **68**, 69
    Sizzling Asian Shrimp 78, **79**
Sizzling Asian Shrimp 78, **79**

Sloppy Joe 149
smoothies 15, 201
    breakfast **22**, 23–25, **24**, 32
snacks, healthy 9–10, 174, **175**
Sorbet Ice Pops, Strawberry 216, **217**
soups
    One-Bowl Meal 133
    Ten-Minute Chicken Noodle Soup 115
spaghetti
    Bacon and Tomato Spaghetti Sauce
        104
    Fresh Tomato Sauce for Spaghetti 98
    Hidden Vegetable Spaghetti
        Bolognese 91
Spicy Potato Wedges 6
steak
    Teriyaki Beef Skewers 142, **143**
steaming 36
sticker charts 8
Sticky BBQ Ribs 146, **147**
Sticky Chicken 122
Sticky Toffee Pudding Cakes 197
stir-fries 36
    Salmon on a Stick with Stir-fried
        Noodles 70, **71**
strawberries
    Strawberries and Cream (smoothie)
        24, 25
    Strawberry Sorbet Ice Pops 216, **217**
sugar, hidden 15
Sunflower Seed, Oat, and Apple Muffins
    183
Sunshine Smoothie **22**, 23
Super Salmon Wrap 67
Swedish Meatballs 145
Sweet Pepper and Tomato Sauce,
    Chicken in 131
sweet potatoes 36
Sweet-and-sour Fish 86

tartar sauce 81
Ten-Minute Chicken Noodle Soup 115
Teriyaki Beef Skewers 142, **143**
toffee
    Apples with Toffee Sauce 203
    Sticky Toffee Pudding Cakes 197
    toffee-banana topping 29
tofu
    Grace's Dairy-Free Summer Berry
        Smoothie 25
Tomato Balsamic Dressing 58
tomatoes
    Annabel's Secret Tomato Sauce 45
    Bacon and Tomato Spaghetti Sauce
        104
    Chicken Balls in Tomato Sauce 132
    Chicken Paillard with Arugula and

Cherry Tomatoes **126**, 127
    Chicken in Tomato and Sweet Pepper
        Sauce 131
    Fresh Tomato Sauce for Spaghetti 98
    Marina's Pasta with Pesto and
        Cherry Tomatoes 97
    Pasta with Tomato and Mascarpone
        Sauce **94**, 95
    Sloppy Joe 149
tortillas
    Vegetable Quesadillas 50, **51**
    Yummy Chicken Quesadillas 128,
        129–30
    see also wraps
Trail Mix Bars 174, **175**
Tropical Fruit Salad 204
Tropical Pops 216
tuna 66
    Tuna Melt Fish Cakes 72

Ultimate Chocolate Cupcakes 190, 191

Vanilla Cupcakes 171
Vegetable Chips 60
Vegetable Kebabs 54
Vegetable Quesadillas 50, **51**
vegetables
    growing your own 36
    hidden 36, 91
    recipes 35–63
vitamin A 21
vitamin B$_{12}$ 21
vitamin C 19, 204, 207
vitamin D 21
vitamin E 21

weaning 9
Wheat-Free Birthday Cake 170–71
wheat-free recipes 151–71
white sauce 75
whole-grain cereals 19
wraps
    Annabel's Tasty Shrimp Wrap 67
    breakfast 32, **33**
    Chinese Chicken Wraps 112, **113**
    Lara's Chicken Wraps 114–15
    Super Salmon Wrap 67

yogurt
    Annabel's Berry Mess **206**, 207
    Yogurt "Pot" Cupcakes 182
Yummy Chicken Quesadillas 128, **129–30**
Yummy Vegetable and Cashew Nut
    Burgers 38, **39**

zinc 21
Zucchini Sticks, Cheesy 46

about the author

ANNABEL KARMEL is a leading author on cooking for children. After the tragic loss of her first child, who died of a rare viral disease at just three months, she wrote her first book, *The Healthy Baby Meal Planner*, which is now an international best seller. Annabel has written fifteen more best-selling books on feeding children, including *Top 100 Baby Purees*, *Favorite Family Meals*, *Complete Party Planner*, and *Lunch Boxes and Snacks*. The mother of three, she is an expert at creating tasty and nutritious meals that children like to eat without the need for parents to spend hours in the kitchen. Annabel writes regularly for national newspapers and is a familiar face on British television as an expert on children's nutritional issues.

In the UK, Annabel has her own line of foods in supermarkets based on her popular recipes for children. She has a line of feeding utensils designed to help babies progress from first tastes to feeding themselves, as well as a line of equipment for preparing and storing baby food, and produces cooking sets for children to have fun in the kitchen and learn to cook. She was awarded an MBE (Member of the British Empire) by the Queen in 2006 for her work in the field of child nutrition.

Annabel travels frequently to the United States. She has appeared on many TV programs, including *Live with Regis and Kelly*, the *Today* show, *The View*, *The Early Show*, and *The Tony Danza Show*. She has also written for leading parenting publications, including parenting.com and babycenter.com.

For more recipes and advice, please visit www.annabelkarmel.com, or download the Annabel Karmel: Baby and Toddler Recipes app.